The Stealth Killer

The Stealth Killer

Is Oral Spirochetosis the
Missing Link in the Dental and
Heart Disease Labyrinth?

By **William D. Nordquist, BS, DMD, MS**

Edited By **Connie Strasheim** *and*
Rebecca Nordquist

BioMed Publishing Group

BioMed Publishing Group
P.O. Box 9012
South Lake Tahoe, CA 96158
www.BioMedPublishers.com

Copyright 2009 by William Nordquist
ISBN 10: 0-9763797-8-3
ISBN 13: 978-0-9763797-8-2

For our other books and DVDs, visit www.biomedpublishers.com.

**Visit Dr. Nordquist online at www.niceteeth.tv, and follow his most
current research at www.biomedpublishers.com/nordquist.**

Disclaimer

This book is not intended as medical advice. It is also not intended to prevent, diagnose, treat or cure disease. Instead, the book is intended only to share the author's research, as would an investigative journalist. The book is provided for informational and educational purposes only, not as treatment instructions for any disease. Much of the book is a statement of opinion in areas where the facts are controversial or do not exist.

If you have a medical problem, please consult a licensed physician; this book is not a substitute for professional medical care. The statements in this book have not been evaluated by the FDA.

Acknowledgements

This work is dedicated to my loving and untiring wife, Yaeko, who helped with the research and emotionally supported me with her dedication during the long hours of writing this book.

Table of Contents

"This book presents a compelling hypothesis. There is a long-established relationship between neurological symptoms and systemic spirochete illness such as syphilis. We also know that oral bacteria are capable of entering systemic circulation.

"Given these facts, it is quite plausible that oral spirochetes can enter the bloodstream and have significant cardiovascular and neurological consequences.

"More research, and funding, is needed to verify these effects, but Dr. Nordquist's book offers an important first step by presenting a systematic articulation of the theory as well as the current state of the evidence."

—Sanjai Rao, M.D.
Assistant Clinical Professor of Psychiatry
University of California, San Diego
Veteran's Hospital, La Jolla, CA

About the Author

Dr. William Nordquist is committed to excellence and has practiced dentistry in San Diego, California, since 1973. He received his Bachelor of Science in chemistry from the Rochester Institute of Technology (RIT) and worked for Eastman Kodak Company as an organic chemist. He received his Doctorate of Dental Medicine (DMD) and Master of Science from the University of Louisville. His Master of Science thesis and research produced many publications relating to surface chemistry of dental enamel and powdered and blocks of fluoro and hydroxyapatite (HA). He completed a general practice residency at the San Diego Naval Regional Medical Center and achieved the rank of lieutenant commander before leaving the Navy and setting up his private practice of dentistry in San Diego in 1976. He is a fellow in the American Academy of Implant Dentistry (AAID) and a diplomat in the American Board of Oral Implantology/Implant Dentistry (ABOI). Dr. Nordquist was named the *2008 International Dentist of the Year* by the American Academy of Implant Dentistry.

Dr. Nordquist is performing ongoing research and a webpage has been created to allow you to follow his work. On this page you will find videos and updates from Dr. Nordquist. The content is easy to access and provides an excellent supplement to this book. To follow Dr. Nordquist's work, visit:

www.biomedpublishers.com/nordquist

Dr. Nordquist's Dental Practice:
Implant Dentistry of San Diego
2304 6th Avenue
San Diego, California 92101
(619) 236-7959
www.niceteeth.tv

Autobiography: A Lifetime of Experience that Set the Stage and Led to the Theories Presented in this Book

When I commiserate over the earlier years of my life, I realize that a disability I have, along with key parts of my life, influenced the way I learned to think. Learning to overcome this disability, along with life experiences that I will present in the next few paragraphs, allowed me to take many seemingly unrelated pieces of knowledge and correlate them into a theory. This theory explains, among other things, how many debilitating chronic diseases, with one initiating cause, become stealth killers after many years of dormant coexistence in our body's tissue.

As a kid, I was an undiagnosed dyslexic. Reading was impossible for me, and I found myself cut off from my classmates because I simply couldn't read. Whenever I attempted to do so, I became so embarrassed that I refused to participate in the lessons. During first and second grades, my desk was moved from the rows where the other kids sat to the front of the classroom near the door so I would be isolated from my classmates. I fell into a pattern that is common to other dyslexics in this situation. Since I was not participating in classwork, I would either daydream or think about funny things to say to amuse my classmates. I would thus entertain them, which would annoy my teacher. As a consequence, I made many trips to the principal's office and was further secluded when the principal sent me to the corner of an empty kitchen behind the refrigerator for punishment.

During those difficult years and as a result of being isolated, I learned to use my mind to amuse myself. I got great pleasure out of philosophizing and theorizing about things that I felt no one had ever contemplated. The serendipity of it all is that I learned at an early age to use my mind to visualize problems and solutions. However, even though this developed ability became important to me in later years; it didn't help me at the time. I got so far behind in my classwork that I flunked third grade. To add insult to injury, my sister, Ellen, who was two years younger than me, skipped third grade, and from then on, until we both finished high school, she and I remained at the same grade level.

My sister thrived in grammar school while I was passed along, year after year, without learning basic reading and writing until seventh grade. In this school system, seventh grade marked the big jump into junior high school. And guess what? By that time, I still couldn't read. In an English class during those first days of junior high school, my teacher asked me to read out loud and realized, during a roar of laughter by my classmates, that I wasn't able to do so. I was sent for special reading instruction and somehow learned enough to continue junior high school in regular classes, along with the other students. I do not know what caused my later success in life, except that I had to work extremely hard to overcome my disability. I distinctly remember my father telling me that my grandfather worked harder than two men. I determined at an early age that if my grandfather could work harder than two men, then I was willing to work three times harder than anyone else to achieve my goals. Going the "third extra mile" has made me tenuous in my pursuit of knowledge and understanding in everything I do. I leave no stone unturned when researching a subject and these are skills that I have needed for my investigation.

Somehow, I managed to achieve good enough grades in high school, and I had a good *basso profundo* deep bass singing voice, which allowed me to get accepted into the Eastman School of Music. I enjoyed music, but ran into a problem when, during the rigors of transitioning my voice from gospel to opera, something happened to my voice. To this day I do not know exactly what happened, but I assume that the strain of trying to sing the high notes necessary in most baritone solos caused me to strain or damage my vocal cords. Today, many years later, my speaking voice still has a slight rasp to it. My voice was never the same after that, and as a result, I was led away from music to chemistry.

I found I could get an A in chemistry. Once I discovered the pleasure of good grades (from chemistry) and experienced a great feeling of accomplishment as a result, I strove to get as many A's as possible.

Rochester Institute of Technology, the school I attended for chemistry, was instrumental in my development as an innovator and a problem solver. RIT was supported by Eastman Kodak Company and was considered to be an excellent training program for the industry.

I was fortunate because I was accepted into the prestigious coop program that alternated school quarters at RIT with work quarters at the synthetic chemistry division of Eastman Kodak Company. Not only did this company pay well and have great employee benefits, but I was also able to work in an area where I learned organic chemistry backward and forward. In the first quarters of my coop program, my first job was in large-scale production of chemicals for color film manufacturing as well as in small-scale production of chemicals for outside sales of chemicals through the outlet called Eastman Organic Chemicals. During the last two quarters of my coop program at Kodak, I performed many of the trouble-shooting jobs for the department. Somehow, I had a knack and insight for problem solving in problematic production procedures. During these last two quarters, I did the trouble-shooting jobs for the synthetic chemistry department.

Since I was efficient in job completion and time management, I always had time left over at the end of my working quarter to perform research. All of the chemical production jobs I did during my work quarters at Kodak required both quality control in production and had time limits to complete each individual job. If I could do the job in less time than the procedure protocol required, then I could save this time for the end of the quarter. I would usually have one to two weeks of time saved up at the end of the quarter before I had to return to the school quarter. Kodak allowed me to use this saved time to pursue my school research projects while I was still employed in my industrial laboratory job. The use of the unlimited facilities at Kodak definitely enhanced my research experience during my undergraduate training. As a result, problem solving and research became my strong suits and would immensely benefit me during the remaining years of my education and dentistry career, as well as provide me with the skills that I would need for finding and piecing together the valuable clues of the dental-heart disease labyrinth. My industrial experience that required performing complex multistep chemical synthesis, higher mathematics, and the ability to see through the complexity of these chemical syntheses to the final finished products, I believe was instrumental in the development of my problem solving pre-dental-medical education.

Kodak tried to recruit me as an undergraduate chemist into the job I had had there. However, I wanted to get a Ph.D. in chemistry. As I applied for Ph.D. programs in chemistry, the military draft status for graduate students changed from 2S (student deferment) to 1A (prime drafting status). I didn't want to be drafted and go to Vietnam, so I changed careers. Medicine, dentistry and veterinarian medicine were the only student deferments remaining. I researched dentistry and found that the field of dental research was wide open and intriguing, so I chose dentistry. My grades and recommendations from Kodak were helpful in my acceptance into dental school.

The late sixties transitional time in dental history, from old-style stand-up dentistry to modern sit-down four-handed dentistry that used dental assistants, certainly benefited me in that the University of Louisville was one of these sites selected by the government for a new dental school. Also, both the medical and dental schools built modern research facilities at the same time. When, during my admissions interview at Louisville, the dental faculty found out about my undergraduate background in chemistry research and development, they immediately began to recruit me into their new DMD-MS research program.

The combined DMD with a post-doctorate MS in oral biology, with a major in oral pathology were extremely beneficial in providing me with an education on oral disease, which subsequently allowed me to develop the theory for this book. Half of my MS didactic courses in dental school were in oral pathology, while the other half were in general pathology at the medical school. As part of my general pathology training, I attended tumor board diagnostic treatment planning sessions with physicians and even assisted in autopsies for one summer. Understanding medicine in general—since dentistry is a part of medicine and not an isolated entity unto itself—was an extremely important part of my training that made it possible for me to understand the relationship between dental and heart disease. I felt this combination of instruction cross-trained me in both dentistry and medicine and provided a rare educational opportunity that isn't found even in today's dental curriculum.

I received a research grant and stipend that allowed me to pursue research in the prevention of tooth decay using various fluorides.

This stipend paid my tuition, books, room, board, research equipment, secretary and full use of the research facility at the University of Louisville School of Dentistry and Medicine.

I still had to take all of the dental school courses, however, including periodontics (the study of gum disease). Periodontics was difficult for me, but I didn't realize why at the time. This is something I have discovered only in recent years, but what I was taught in periodontics back then didn't make sense to me. After achieving high grades during my first two years of medical and dental didactic courses, I got straight Cs in my periodontal courses, which didn't help my grade point average in the clinical third and fourth years of my training. This fact beset me for many years and only recently, after doing the research for this book, do I have a much better understanding of the full implications and complexity of periodontal disease.

The research I completed at Louisville resulted in several professional articles that were published in four major dental research journals. I was also invited to speak at the International Association of Dental Research and to members of the National Institute of Health. From early on in my career, I became accustomed to lecturing and dealing with dentists from the highest ranks. The knowledge that sodium and stannous fluoride inhibit bacterial growth had been cemented into my early memory during my research days, and these fluorides are used in toothpaste today to help prevent dental disease. Later I will tell you how I use these two fluorides in preventing recurrent periodontal disease.

The intensity of concurrently attending dental and graduate school caused me to feel as though my clinical skills were lacking; therefore, I joined the United States Navy and entered its hospital residence program for one year in San Diego. I further practiced on a submarine tender, USS *Sperry AS-12*, during my second and third years. I achieved the rank of lieutenant commander. These were great years, and I increased my skills in general and surgical dentistry. The surgical training gave me the confidence later to pursue implant dentistry. Being involved in implant dentistry served as a catalyst to investigate the reasons why infections cause dental implants to fail. As a young lieutenant dentist, and because of my research background, I was honored to lecture in continuing education seminars. After the Navy, I set up a general dentistry practice in San Diego and have been practicing there ever since.

Introduction

This book describes the relationship between dental periodontal (gum) disease and heart disease, as well as other systemic inflammatory diseases, including Alzheimer's and other plaque-forming neurological diseases, diabetes, premature birth, autoimmune diseases, and cancer. The relationship between dental and heart disease has been reported in scientific literature and national news for several years; however, an understanding of, or probable theories as to why these relationships exist have been absent. Ever since the surgeon general of the United States published a report on the relationship between periodontal and heart disease in 2000, I have been studying this subject with intensity and interest. My first illustration in this book, a chart showing the expenditures for the top five most costly health conditions in the United States for 2000 and 2004 (Figure A, next page), provides insights into the economic magnitude and implications of the subject of this book, for reasons that will become evident later. Heart disease is the most expensive disease to treat, followed by mental disorders and cancer. Health-care expenditures and lost productivity as a result of death and disability because of cardiovascular disease are projected to be $394 billion in 2005[1]. Three of the five conditions in the chart—namely, heart disease, cancer, and mental disorders—may be all related to a specific oral bacterial condition. This condition, caused by a single microorganism, could be a major contributory factor in health conditions that cost the health-care system more than $204.2 billion in 2004 and nearly $1 trillion for the five-year period ending 2003.

Aetna Insurance Company[2] performed a study on its clients who carried both dental and medical insurance coverage under its policies. This study examined whether periodontal treatment can contribute to changes in overall risk and medical expenditures for three chronic conditions specifically: diabetes, coronary heart

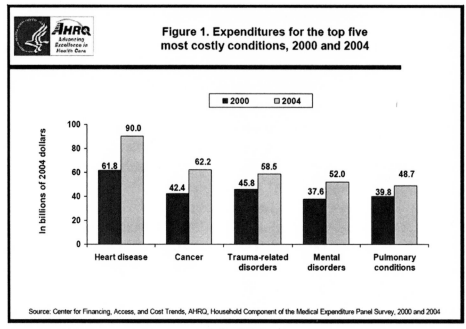

FIGURE A
Expenditures for the top five most costly conditions, 2000 and 2004.

disease, and/or cerebrovascular disease. The results were asto-nishing. The patients who had these three conditions and who were also being treated for periodontal disease had drastically higher per member, per month medical expenses than those members who did not have periodontal disease. The findings suggest that periodontal treatment (a proxy for the presence of periodontal disease) impacts the per member, per month costs for these three chronic conditions. In other words, people with periodontal disease cost the insurance industry, Medicare, and the fee-for-service paying public billions of dollars. Periodontal disease is turning out to be a far greater health problem than any health professional could have imagined.

Once it's contracted by patients, cures for these conditions are elusive, almost impossible to treat effectively, and expensive.

What's more, the cost of treatment is bankrupting the Medicare system and dramatically increasing the cost of health care and insurance. There is no hope for curing these diseases, only for successful treatment of their symptoms. Even though cures are not likely, most, if not all, of these conditions can be prevented with education, along with simple treatment and inexpensive home-care remedies that are monitored by a dentist.

The theory I present regarding the relationship between dental and heart disease is the result of eight years of study. The first years were frustrating and unproductive for me; however, March of 2007 began a remarkable year of discovery. I discovered two key clues while watching the PBS documentary, *The Modern Epidemic: Heart Disease in America*[3]. This began my journey through a trail of more than 100 years of evidence to discover a convincing theory that would link gum disease to atherosclerotic heart disease, as well as other systemic diseases including Alzheimer's, pancreatic, and stomach cancer, and many more chronic inflammatory diseases.

The documentary, produced by Elizabeth Arledge, detailed the heart disease epidemic in America. Even before watching this documentary, I knew that periodontal disease, or gum disease, was related to heart disease. Most dentists have been aware of this fact for years and many professional journals have been reporting on the relationship for at least fifteen years. The public is also somewhat aware of the relationship; however, up until now, no specific mechanism or identification of the main culprit that links the two has ever been found. Only those who have performed epidemiological studies have speculated about it. No one has known whether there is a cause-and-effect relationship between the diseases or whether they have been coincidentally found together when people get sick or die. Did dental periodontal disease cause heart disease, or were they both a result of something else?

I was engrossed in the documentary, especially when the film-maker documented a new ultrasound device able to diagnose 99 percent more atherosclerotic lesions than could previously be found with older angiogram methods for detection of atherosclerotic plaques. That patients have a much greater number of lesions than previously thought, as evidenced by the documentary, was clue No. 1 for me to begin a new line of research. I thought, What is capable of causing all those plaques and how are they related to gum disease? This disturbing fact created great urgency within me to discover why there were so many plaques, and if these were in some way related to periodontal disease.

The second fact that struck me about the documentary was its mention of heart disease as a modern epidemic, since it was only after World War II that people started to "drop dead" with heart attacks in great numbers. Why? My thoughts scrambled through what I knew about heart disease, leaving me in a quandary that quickly morphed into enthusiasm to find an answer. I distinctly remember a sense of destiny that beleaguered me as I continued to watch the program. Since that evening, I have been constantly reminded of the poignant words contained within the program, "Every minute someone dies of heart disease."

As I continued to watch the documentary, I waited for the film-maker to mention the relationship between heart and gum disease, but the 90-minute documentary ended without even a word on the subject. Fortunately, talk-show host Larry King had followed the program with a panel of experts who then discussed the documentary. Near the end of their conversation, Dr. Michael Roizen, from the Cleveland Clinic Foundation, said, "Do some easy things for your health...flossing your teeth prevents periodontal disease...one of the leading causes of heart disease is inflammation in the blood vessels, and for some reason periodontal disease causes that. We don't know why." In the end, those few words comprised all that was mentioned regarding the relationship between periodontal and heart disease. Why?

It was 11 p.m. when the program finished and I ran upstairs to tell my wife, Yaeko, that we were going to Los Angeles the following weekend to visit the medical library at University of California, Los Angeles. I told her about the documentary and why I needed to find a solution to the dental-heart disease problem. The next afternoon, I outlined a simple theory concerning the relationship between dental and heart disease.

I spent the next two weekends at the library. After the first weekend, I had accumulated a stack of articles, and based on what I had learned, I realized I needed to investigate older literature. In a library across campus, I checked out several old bacteriology and periodontal disease textbooks.

Ironically, I had planned on taking a two-week writing vacation in April 2007 in Cabo San Lucas, Mexico. I needed to write several papers on implant dentistry cases that I had collected over the years. These were seemingly unrelated to my current research and concerned infections around dental implants. I had not had time to review most of the articles and books I had collected at the library before leaving on my trip, so I had no idea what was in store.

During the first week, I worked ten to twelve hours every day writing five papers describing infection associated with dental implants. One paper reported on the relationship between root canal–treated teeth and foci of infection (a small pocket of infection) associated with these teeth, as well as on infection and bone loss around adjacent dental implants. Another paper I had to write concerned a case of periodontal infection that had occurred within three months of placing three implants and had resulted in bone loss where there had been no prior sign of gum infection. Yet another paper dealt with a long and difficult search for the source of an infection in a patient whose infection was draining from the bottom of a single implant. What was interesting about these studies was that all of them dealt with oral infection associated with dental implants—information that would give me insight into the problem I had come here to solve. My first week in Cabo, I didn't know that the papers I had originally gone there to write would be associated with the bacteria I would later implicate and write about during my second week there. That is, those that would ultimately link periodontal disease to the specific mechanism that leads to heart disease, as well as other chronic inflammatory diseases mentioned earlier.

I began reading all of the professional articles and textbooks I had brought with me from the UCLA library and began to realize the magnitude of what I was finding in the literature. Combined with what I had written the week before, I put together the first draft of this book, which describes the relationship between dental and heart disease.

Within a few weeks after my return to San Diego, I was introduced to Dr. Alan MacDonald's research on Lyme disease. MacDonald is a medical doctor, general pathologist and researcher, and has published some of the best breakthrough information I have ever read on Lyme disease, which is caused by bacteria similar to that which causes gum disease. Over the next few months, due in part to what I learned from MacDonald and other resources, other pieces of the puzzle would fall into place. Even a few weeks prior to the final cut-off date for writing this book, I continued to make important discoveries. Despite all I learned, this work is yet ongoing and more discoveries are needed to verify fully the information in this book. The past twelve months have been the most interesting and productive months of my life. My hope is that, in the future, this research will help to prevent periodontal, heart and other related diseases. People who already have these diseases need a major break-through in treatment. Now that a rational explanation for their cause has been theorized, we can begin looking for a cure.

How Bacteria Influenced My Early Dental Practice

Oral bacteria started to affect my life in the early eighties, soon after I began my dental career. It all started when a patient I had treated for gum disease, and upon whom I had used traditional surgical means along with methods of hygiene, relapsed within two years. This patient was also a smoker; however, at the time, the injurious effects of smoking upon dental and medical health had not yet been fully established. This patient, as is the case with many who have gum disease, did not follow up with regular cleanings at my office after I treated his gum disease with periodontal surgery. After he left my practice (possibly thinking he had been cured by the surgery) he found that after only two years, his signs and symptoms of gum disease had returned. He sought treatment for his relapsed periodontal disease at a local periodontal specialist's office. This periodontist, who happened to be an influential past president of the local periodontal society, had practiced in San Diego for almost fifty years, and performed a second full-mouth surgery on this patient. Within a short time, the disease reoccurred, and the patient relapsed yet once again, thus necessitating a third surgery. At this point, the patient was beginning to get suspicious about the number of surgeries that were required for him in such a short interval of time, and asked the periodontist why he needed three surgeries. The well-known and respected periodontist was taken aback by the question and informed the patient that he had only performed two surgeries. The patient corrected him and told him I had also performed periodontal surgery on him before he had come to his office. The periodontist's reaction was, "If Dr. Nordquist had performed the surgery right in the first place, I would not be doing it for a third time again today." Little did either one of us know at the time the contents of this book. That was my first traumatic litigious event as a young dentist, and the blame I received was directly related to ignorance in dentistry of the actual cause of, and the adequate treatment for, periodontal disease.

During those early years, I performed my own hygiene cleanings for patients, which I found to be boring and tedious. From the early 1980s until 1992, I turned over teeth cleanings and the nonsurgical treatment of periodontal disease to a hygienist and shifted my concentration to other areas of dentistry, including orthodontics, prosthetics, crown, bridge and dental implants. In 1992, I sold my general practice in San Diego's east county, and for five years, I limited my practice to implant dentistry in my new downtown office. My implant dentistry patients came from a marketing program that attracted, for the most part, patients who did not have a regular dentist or who did not visit their dentist on a regular basis. Those who did have regular dentists sought implant treatment from me since their dentist didn't place implants. These patients usually had multiple missing teeth, most of which had been lost due to periodontal disease. Before placing any dental implants, however, I would perform whatever periodontal treatment on these patients I thought was necessary. Implant failures from such patients who were not under the regular care of a dentist have provided invaluable clues over the years.

Implant dentistry has completely changed dentistry by providing better treatment options for patients when they lose their teeth. Dentists have traditionally treated spaces in the mouth caused by missing teeth with dental bridges and partial dentures. With the advent of implant dentistry, missing teeth are now replaced by titanium screws that fit into the jawbone and that have teeth attached to them. Most dentists doing implants today report a ten-year success rate approaching 95 percent.

For many years, I have had the opportunity to serve as an expert witness in malpractice litigation. Almost every lawsuit I have been involved in, whether I was serving as an expert witness for the defendant or plaintiff, or as the defendant, the specific bacteria discussed in this book had something to do with the unfavorable outcome of the implant case, in one way or another. The elusiveness and complexity of the organisms involved in periodontal disease leaves clinicians vulnerable to lawsuits, especially in the area of implant dentistry. Implant dentistry is the ob-gyn of dentistry, meaning that implant dentists are being sued as much as ob-gyn doctors. Fear of getting sued is the dread of implant dentists. Many dental malpractice insurance companies have discontinued coverage of dental implants because of the number of lawsuits brought against those dentists who place dental implants. Even though the literature and most experienced implant dentists confirm they have an approximate 95 percent success rate with dental implants, the remaining 5 percent of failed implants cause so many lawsuits that many implant dentists question the wisdom of working in this vulnerable area of dentistry. Many dentists quit practicing dentistry altogether as a result.

The disproportionate amount of energy that has been required to solve the infection problems of those few failed cases, however, has resulted in extremely positive outcomes. Major discoveries concerning the treatment of gum disease have arisen from such adversities. In my case, without the severe criticism I received from my dentistry colleagues, I would never have scrutinized the bacteria problem close enough to be able to discover the relationship between these organisms and heart disease. The principles I discuss in this book should eliminate most of the litigation problems if clinicians understand the almost impossible bacterial milieu we deal with. As a result of dentists' understanding and ability to treat periodontal disease, ultimately, the public will benefit by paying lower fees for dentistry, which will in turn save millions of dollars in health-care costs and reduced medical insurance premiums. And in the end, experts in dental malpractice will not have any basis for criticism, as infections occurring around dental implants will then be explainable, treatable, and possibly eliminated. Infection around dental implants can become a legal moot point.

I purchased my first microscope in 2001 and a research-grade microscope in 2007. After studying the plaque samples of patients with differing degrees of periodontal disease, I became as confused as one could possibly become. Medical literature is full of studies in culturing bacteria; however, there exists scant information on the appearance of live bacteria as they are seen under the microscope. Further, it is even more rare to find literature that correlates the microscopic appearance of bacteria with the cultured studies of these same bacteria. Throughout the first few years of my studies, I used to tell patients I had no idea what I was seeing on the live microscopic slides of the bacteria samples I had taken from their mouths.

As the years passed, with the help of Bill Lauders, a microbiologist and owner of the hygiene and microscope supply company Oratec Inc., I began to understand some of what I was seeing. I had told patients that because of the severe implications of heart disease and diabetes and because periodontal disease–causing bacteria were somehow related to these conditions, it was important for me to study and treat their periodontal bugs—bacteria observed at 1000 power look like little pond bugs. Diseased areas of the mouth have bacteria that show various degrees of movement. The worse the disease is, the faster and more furious the motion of the bacteria. Also I learned that certain bacteria, especially spirochetes, are marker bacteria for what I consider to be severe disease. Based on research done by Drs. Paul Keyes and

Daniel Watt, I subsequently began to treat patients who had "mobile" bacteria. Through my studies, I learned that normal flora in plaque is quiet and non-motile.

The learning process is never ending. What I have learned up until now will no doubt provide me with an even greater understanding later. Meanwhile, in the next chapter, I will begin discussing the elements that form the hypotheses for the relationship between dental and heart disease.

Chapter 1
A Paradigm Shift in the Way I Understood Gum Disease and Its Relationship to Heart Disease

This opening statement is written by Dr. Richard Ellen—considered the world authority on oral spirochetes—from the University of Toronto, in his professional publication titled, *Spirochetes at the Forefront of Periodontal Infection.4*

- *"What if a group of microorganisms emerged subgingivally (under the gums) at a much higher population density during the onset of inflammatory lesions (infections) than detectable in healthy sites in severely diseased periodontium (gum tissue) and their presence correlated with progressive periodontal (gum) disease activity?"*

- *What if their population was reduced when standard therapy was given, but their numbers remained significant in other instances where they had developed resistance to treatment?*

- *What if they were tissue- invasive (and had the ability in get into the body's cells themselves)?*

- *What if they selectively evaded or suppressed key pathways of local immunity?*

- *What if they were highly proteolytic (able to digest protein), produced noxious (poisonous) metabolites, and surface proteins that disabled cell cytoskeletal dynamics (which refers to the ability of the cell to defend itself) and which control cellular migration and chemotaxis?*

The answer: Infectious disease specialists such as periodontists would target such a group of microorganisms for intensive investigation and translate their findings into informative texts for health practitioners and the public at large. As a group of bacteria, and in some cases, as individual species, oral spirochetes satisfy all of the above postulates that would categorize them as "periodontal pathogens," but unfortunately, get very little respect from the research community and generate very little attention among the practicing community of dentists. Why?"

How did we get to this sad state of affairs? Ellen laments the lack of urgency among clinical dentists to diagnose and treat this proven pathogen, which is the most likely candidate for causing the most virulent form of periodontal disease. My postulate discussed later in the book that bacteria can evade the immune system correlates with evidence found in Ellen's professional paper, which demonstrates that oral spirochetes may not only be able to evade the immune system from the onset of their presence in the body, but also, once attacked, may be able to hijack the immune system and use it as a vital component of their lifecycle.

The above quote is appropriate for the beginning paragraph of the book because it demonstrates there are researchers who are beginning to put the pieces of the puzzle together. However, practicing dental clinicians do not understand much of this research, or if, in the unlikely scenario, they do, they are not incorporating this knowledge into their practices.

My periodontal training and understanding of periodontal disease are typical of what is found in dentistry today. Like so many dentists, I frankly haven't understood it, but have treated the disease the best I knew how. Brushing and flossing and three- to six-month follow-up hygiene appointments have been the treatment norms and what I have practiced. In my experience, as long as patients have followed this regimen, they have appeared to be normal. I now know I have been only maintaining—not curing—periodontal disease. When patients were negligent and didn't follow up on care, or didn't remember to schedule follow-up visits to see me, the disease always returned. Whenever these patients would return to my office years later, their periodontal disease would be worse than before. If I performed periodontal (gum) surgery on a patient the way I was trained to do in dental school, a large percentage would relapse and need further surgery only two or three years later. It was very discouraging, and eventually, I turned to non-surgical treatment with better results, although not always. Of course, whenever relapses would occur, unfortunately, we always blamed the patient for not brushing his or her teeth properly. But we could not explain why patients who never brushed their teeth did not get periodontal disease. Was brushing and flossing effective against the disease? Apparently not.

In 2000, I attended an implant dentistry seminar in Biloxi, Mississippi, where I was introduced to Watt, who worked with Keyes of the National Institute of Health. Keyes first discovered the bacteria called streptococcus mutans, which causes tooth decay. With the use of a microscope, he also discovered that non-surgical techniques were just as effective as surgical ones for the treatment of periodontal disease when working with highly compliant patients. Many general dentists, but not the majority of periodontists, embrace this concept. Thus, a thirty-year controversy regarding the surgical (for the most part performed by periodontists) and non-surgical (predominately performed by general dentists) treatment of gum disease was born. Later in this book, I will address this controversy. As it turns out, both perspectives had merit.

At this implant dentistry meeting, I discussed with Watt the meaning of the 2000 Surgeon General Report concerning the relationship between dental and heart disease. It was during this discussion that I decided to change course in my dental practice. I purchased my first microscope, and Watt was instrumental in helping me to set up a new non-surgical periodontal program for my patients using this new microscope. I coined the program Life Guard, since I felt that by treating periodontal disease in this manner, I would be saving my patients' lives. At that time, I didn't understand the full implications of the program. Today, I definitely know I am saving lives.

For many years, almost from the very beginning of my thirty-plus years of dental practice, I was aware of those few dentists from around the country who did have microscopes; however, they were ridiculed, and they were not taken seriously. Again, the lines were drawn between the periodontist who didn't advocate microscopes and the few general dentists who embraced their use. This time, the microscope advocates won the controversy.

Many dentists and hygienists have also used microscopes as a scare tactic to motivate their patients to brush and floss their teeth better, but have not used them necessarily as a diagnostic tool for deciding upon different modes of treatment for their patients. Prior to my investigations, I did not think I needed the microscope because I believed I could diagnosis and treat periodontal disease in the traditional way I had been taught in dental school. So, for the first ten years of my practice, I treated gum disease traditionally, with deep scaling and root planing and surgery, including by teaching patients good hygiene. Regrettably, these patients always seemed to relapse and would need another surgery within two to five years.

Since I have been converted to one of those "dentists with a microscope," thanks to Watt, I have undertaken the quest of solving the mystery of the relationship between gum and heart disease. For seven years, I studied the microbiology of bacteria from each and every one of my periodontally diseased patients. At first, it was frustrating looking at bacteria I knew absolutely nothing about. Even the microbiologist experts didn't know the actual names of the oral bacteria I saw under the microscope. Bacteria that can be cultured by microbiologists have traditional Latin names; however, bacteria observed under the microscope don't have names, except by basic description, including "mobile rods" and "spinning rods" or various sizes of spirochetes: "small," "medium," and "large." The bacteria I observed under my microscope were many, and, over the years, trying to guess what they were made it difficult to continue studying them. However, I was tenacious, and I plodded along, year after year, patient after patient, despite not knowing what in the world I was looking at under the microscope.

There are approximately six hundred different bacteria in the mouth. The treatments I gave to my patients once I learned about all of these bacteria was based on the number of different bacteria I found, their relative mobility, and whether they included spirochetes. During the early years of this project, when I found what I thought was disease, I would take the bacteria found in the plaque samples and send them to Dr. Jorgen Slots. Slots worked at the Microbiology Testing Laboratory at the University of Southern California and would identify the bacteria and test their sensitivity to antibiotics. Subsequently, I would treat the patient with the recommended antibiotics and follow-up with another examination using the microscope. All too often, there would still be active bacteria present after the recommended treatment had been completed and the patient's disease would not be cured or controlled. For this reason, the microbiology culturing and testing were not adequate for providing the results I needed. My microscope was more accurate, and through its use, I would know when I got a patient's antibiotics right, because there would no longer be any movement of bacteria within the microscopic field. I used this method of diagnosis and treatment until 2007. After that time, I changed my treatment regimen because I found that antibiotics were not effective against certain bacteria, which are the focal subject of this book. Now that I better understand the full implications of the diseases they cause, I treat them more aggressively using a laser, curettage (cleaning out the infected tissue from the "gumline"), and a combination of chemical irrigations.

The following chapters will detail the discoveries I made linking gum disease to atherosclerosis. The literary research I completed follows a 150-year-plus trail of evidence on periodontal and other similar spirochetal diseases, and introduces a very persuasive theory regarding the link between dental disease and heart disease, as well as other chronic plaque-forming inflammatory diseases.

It is important to note that the clues in this investigation were fragmented and, without the suspicion of a possible link between these two diseases, it wouldn't have been possible to decipher the convoluted path that led to the answer to this stealthy riddle. As previously mentioned, heart disease began in relatively recent history, following World War II. I will also present research that has been completed in the past fifteen years linking periodontal and heart disease. If these two diseases are related and periodontal disease causes heart disease, then what changed in periodontal disease 20 to 30 years before World War II that led to the modern heart disease epidemic after World War II? Other questions I will address include: Why is gum disease so easy to transmit? Why are dental and heart disease so evenly disseminated throughout the industrialized world? It seems both are modern epidemics. Why?

With these questions posed, I began researching information, beginning from the mid-1800s. My purpose was twofold: first, to search the periodontal disease literature for a major change in the practice of periodontics that occurred sometime before World War II; and second, to search the bacteriology textbooks to find why periodontal disease is so easily transmissible. I wanted to ascertain whether the organisms that cause gum disease have a lifecycle or transmission vectors that medicine has not yet understood. It is probable I performed this research with an entirely different motive than those who had researched this topic in the past. It is interesting to note that most of the books I reviewed were old archives and hadn't been checked out for at least thirty years, but the pieces of the puzzle were all there. However, without the knowledge of a link that has only recently been revealed, the connection would not have been obvious.

Chapter 2
Understanding the Basic Principles of Atherosclerotic Heart Disease

As I was researching the old literature, I came across a book called *Interstitial Gingivitis or So-called Pyorrhea Alveolaris,* which was published in 1899. Pyorrhea is the old name for gum disease, and alveolaris is the old name for the gingival or gum tissue. Periodontal disease as described in this book is exactly the same as lesions of atherosclerotic heart disease are described today. The lesion is located in a blood vessel next to a tooth, rather than in atherosclerotic plaque in the heart. Also, at the time this book was written, periodontal disease was known to be caused by bacteria found in gum-diseased tissue around teeth.

Studying live *in vivo* tissue from atherosclerotic heart lesions is difficult. If what occurs in the heart is the same disease process as that which occurs in the periodontally diseased mouth as described above, and it seems to be, where better to study atherosclerotic disease than in the mouth where it is easily accessible? Even though there was no evidence as to which specific bacteria caused the atherosclerotic lesion at the time, today, the evidence definitely leads to oral spirochetes.

The old book, an excerpt quoted in the next paragraph, describes what we know today as atherosclerotic heart disease in detail; however, it is noteworthy to observe that the description of the lesion was describing periodontal disease instead that was taken from the gum tissue around diseased periodontally involved teeth. The entire quotation from the old book is located in Appendix I. Following are a few excerpts to illustrate the wisdom and knowledge of Talbot documented so many years ago:

> "**Endarteritis Obliterans:** Endarteritis is an inflammation of the internal coat of an artery or capillary, generally of chronic type. ...Inflammation of the intima of the blood vessels may be due to irritation from without or within. ...The vasa vasorum becomes swollen; the white blood corpuscles crowd into the terminal capillaries and migrate into the extra vascular spaces. Rapid proliferation of the round-cell elements takes place. The walls of the vessels become thickened. ...Under these circumstances a germ disease or other toxins may have an affinity for a certain organ, tissue or part, and produce irritation in the capillaries in a distant part of the body."

The illustration (figures 1 & 2, next page) he presented in his book is exactly what we see today in atherosclerosis.

It's interesting to note that 108 years ago, Talbot described inflammation caused by bacteria that he believed caused a thickening of capillary walls, and that this phenomenon of inflammation could spread to other parts of the body. The evidence presented in this book suggests that bacteria, namely oral spirochetes, travel via the bloodstream to enter the endothelial lining of distal blood vessels where they cause atherosclerotic lesions. A mechanism for this phenomenon will be presented later. In any case, evidence suggests that the bacteria that caused the inflammatory lesions described by Talbot are also the same bacteria found in heart disease. Did Talbot, so many years ago, describe the mechanism for heart disease and its relationship to,

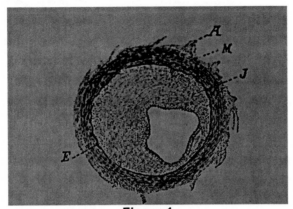

Figure 1
Atherosclerotic lesion taken from Dr. Talbot's book published in 1899.

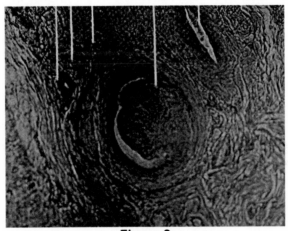

Figure 2
Atherosclerotic lesion from small blood vessel next to inflamed gum
disease next to a tooth in 1899.

or possible origin from, periodontal disease? The lesions found
in both diseases are identical.

Furthermore, atherosclerotic heart disease today can be described in exactly the same terms Talbot used. It is a thickening
of the walls of cardiac arteries to the point where they become

clogged or obstructed so blood flow to the heart muscles is restricted. When this happens, the heart tissue dies and the heart can no longer function properly. Years ago, when there was no understanding of heart disease or treatment regimens, a large number of patients who had heart attacks would die. With modern technology and understanding, today more people who have heart attacks can be saved.

With the foundation now established, an explanation of different types of heart disease and how they develop from periodontal disease (described in laymen terms) is in order at this point. Uncontrolled bacterial colonies living below the gumline in the gingival sulcus (the area between the gums and the teeth) easily gain entrance into the bloodstream via bacteremias (bacteria entering the bloodstream through bleeding gums around the teeth) and cause one of two different types of heart disease:

1. Inflammatory atherosclerotic heart disease. This occurs when mini-abscesses are formed in the endothelial lining of blood vessels and cause plaque formation (or a hardening of the arteries). Through very complicated mechanisms, which are discussed later, these plaques can burst and can cause heart attacks and strokes.

2. Bacterial endocarditis. This is caused by a bacteremia of a virulent strain of streptococcus bacteria that produces an acute infection in the heart. This is a dangerous form of heart disease and can kill a person rapidly. The bloodstream is a fast-moving river of blood. Wherever there are turns or bifurcations in the blood vessels in the heart, turbulence can occur in these areas as little pools of blood form and stagnate. Bacteria from periodontal infections congregate in these stagnant pools and attach to the blood vessels, starting an acute infection. The body then starts to react to this infection with a typical inflammatory response. White blood cells attack

the area and collect on the surface of the heart's arterial wall. The cells normally fight the pathogens and die, but if the immune response continues, more and more deposits build up, clogging the artery. If the condition is left undetected, it can lead to death.

Today, atherosclerotic heart disease is far worse than we ever imagined. The latest method for detecting heart disease uses miniature ultrasound probes that are inserted and guided into the cardiac arteries, and represents a great improvement in diagnosing heart disease. Traditional angiograms only show approximately 1 percent of lesions that are actually present in the blood vessels, when compared to the new miniature intravascular ultrasound methods of diagnosis that show 100 percent of lesions. In a way, however, this new technology is a double-edged sword. On the one hand, it's encouraging in that even the minutest lesions can be discovered; however, it also shows us that heart disease is far worse than anyone had previously thought. Even though the exact mechanism for the relationship between dental and heart disease has not been described, the plethora of periodontal bacteria that have been found in atherosclerotic lesions provides another piece of evidence that the initiating factor for the development of heart disease is bacterial.

The information contained within the previously mentioned PBS television special, *The Hidden Epidemic: Heart Disease in America*[5], provided important clues for dentists. Chilling statistics in this documentary included the following: heart disease now kills half of all Americans; every 26 seconds someone in the United States has a cardiac event; and once every minute, someone dies as a result of cardiac problems/complications. According to Dr. Daniel Levy, the vast majority of us, by the time we've reached a fairly ripe age, have advanced atherosclerosis in our blood vessels. One important point and clue to this is the fact that heart disease is a modern phenomenon that has become an epidemic since World War II.

During a long-term investigation of heart disease, called the Farmington study, 5,209 "average" people were studied over a twenty-year period. After thirteen years, in 1961, the study reported its first findings. Three characteristics that were consistently found among members of the study were that they had high blood pressure, high cholesterol and were smokers. Levy commented on these findings and said that with the emergence of the knowledge of these characteristics, the whole equation in the approach to heart disease changed after 1961. As a result, millions of dollars worth of drugs have been developed and sold to mitigate the above-mentioned symptoms of heart disease; however, the disease has not been cured. These drugs merely treat the symptoms. A new paradigm change in the understanding of heart disease may now occur once again as a result of evidence presented in this book.

Through my studies of inflammatory atherosclerotic heart disease, it became evident to me that the researchers have no idea why atherosclerotic lesions react in the way that they do, as an autoimmune inflammatory process. The lesions seem to be micro-auto-immune disease reactions occurring within the endothelial lining of blood vessels. Richard J Fink, M.D., in his book, *Inflammatory Atherosclerosis: Characteristics of the Injurious Agent*, describes an unknown injurious agent (IA). He believes something is causing the inflammatory immune cell, which is meant to heal the disease, to turn on itself and thereby cause inflammatory atherosclerotic heart disease. How does this happen? Somehow, when the inflammatory cell shows up to react to the IA, it is changed. Once the immune cell attacks the IA, it is somehow transformed and itself becomes the target of the immune system. The whole immune system is turned against itself, thereby creating an autoimmune reaction. From the dentists' perspective, as the atherosclerotic process continues, the lesions produced can best be described as abscesses, a common occurrence produced in the gums as a result of periodontal disease.

Studies that have linked heart disease to periodontal disease have been found in the dental literature for many years[6] [7] [8] [9] [10] [11] [12] [13] [14]. However, these studies were not brought into the public eye until the *Surgeon General Report*[15] published a report on the link between the two diseases in the early 2000s. This is the first and only report produced by the Surgeon General about dentistry in the entire history of governmental reports on medicine. This fact that the Surgeon General took the time to emphasize the relationship between dental and heart disease shows the importance that the government placed on this subject. Bacteria found in periodontal disease have been isolated in the atherosclerotic heart lesion, and dentists and physicians are now seeking the reason as to why this is so.

As periodontal disease is related to atherosclerotic heart disease, the same inflammatory process is related to many other chronic diseases as well. To be discussed later, recent studies have shown that oral bacteria are also present in the human brain and are associated with Alzheimer's disease[16]. Periodontal disease is also related to premature birth, diabetes, and pancreatic cancer.

Finally, if periodontal disease is related to heart disease, or if the bacteria that cause periodontal disease also cause heart disease, what happened or changed in dentistry twenty or thirty years before World War II that could have been a contributing factor to the sudden increase in heart disease today? This is a question that demands an answer.

Chapter 3
Understanding the History of Periodontal Disease, Its Etiology, and Its Many Bacteria

If heart disease is described by some to be a modern hidden epidemic, and if recent research is correct and periodontal disease is related to heart disease, then it makes sense to look back before World War II to discover what has changed about periodontal disease. Based on this premise, I reviewed the old literature to find an answer. So far, we know that that atherosclerosis is a chronic, slow-developing disease. We can assume that it requires several decades to incubate, develop and produce the lesions in the heart that cause heart attacks. So what happened to change the way periodontal disease was viewed, or dentists' understanding thereof or what bacteria had changed that could have led to the drastic increase in heart attacks after War World II?

During my research, articles written in the early 1900s reminded me of Vincent's disease, better known as "Trench Mouth," a predominately spirochetal-fusiform infection that plagued our troops in World War I and which is well known to dentists today. This disease was unique; it started and was reported in the dental and medical literature during the exact predicted window of time in which I surmised that something had changed in periodontal disease. Also, I discovered in the literature many other references that documented common forms of gum disease, some having to do with spirochetes, and which dated back to the mid-18th century. Apparently, these periodontal diseases have been prevalent in humans from the earliest time in history. Articles that I found on this subject included: "Loosening of the Teeth,"[17] "Riggs's disease,"[18] [19] and "Pyorrhoea Alveolaris."[20] [21] The first reference I could find about Vincent's organisms was dated around 1920[22]. Vincent recognized the importance of bacteria known as fusiforms and spirochetes, so in honor of his investigation, an infection was named after him. Vincent's disease, however, was a more virulent type of periodontal disease than was earlier reported before its discovery. The importance of this infection was recognized and its prevalence was obvious based on the large number of articles published on the disease during the two decades following 1920.

As previously mentioned, the information on Vincent's disease was published within the same time frame in which I predicted that something must have changed in the periodontal disease dental literature. The arrival of Vincent's disease, once referred to as Acute Necrotizing Ulcerative Gingivitis (ANUG), and which is now referred to as Necrotizing Ulcerative Gingivitis (NUG), correlates with subsequent infection of the population (after a period of incubation) and the development of heart disease following World War II. In other words, the beginning of the process that led to heart disease would have started at about the time when Vincent's disease was discovered and described.

Oral spirochetal bacteria essentially similar to the spirochetes that populate the gums of most modern people today were also observed and reported in the golden age of microscopy (1880–

1920). Vincent's disease, however, was different and caused acute infection of the gums. This virulent infection actually kills the gum tissue between the teeth, leaving punched-out areas between the teeth where once-healthy gum was located. It is extremely destructive.

What is the significance of this connection? Where did the new strain or the more virulent form of spirochetal bacteria come from? The research needed to discover their origins, as well as the origins of other virulent strains, could take millions of dollars. In addition, it would involve studying the DNA of spirochetes in the mouths of people in diverse populations all over the world. Such studies could be done, but suffice it to say that whatever these virulent spirochetal bacteria are, they were probably introduced into the populations of Europe and migrated to the United States and the remainder of the industrialized world during the early 1900s. Similar to the bacteria that cause syphilis, the populations that were first exposed to these bacteria lacked resistance and fell victim to its destructive mechanisms.

The Harvard professor Socransky[23], while reviewing the historical evidence for periodontal bacteria, noted that the prevalence of Vincent's disease has been declining in many industrialized countries for many decades. He pointed out how common the disease was during 1915–1930. He mentions in his article that a Dr. Daley in Boston found the prevalence of Vincent's disease to be 30 percent of the one thousand patients who had gone to Tufts Dental College at that time for dental treatment. The microscopic pattern and clinical appearance of the bacteria back then were exactly as we describe them today. He also mentions that the disease was rare prior to 1917.

Another point that Socransky makes after reviewing numerous articles written during this time period is that the disease is easily transmitted from one person to another. This coincides with similar data that was reported later using more modern methods of documentation.

Spouses and children[24] [25] [26] of symptomatic patients being treated frequently are found to have the same bacterial patterns and spirochetes in their mouths. By an unknown transmission vector, a new strain of bacteria, possibly fusiform, but definitely spirochetal, was introduced into a population that had various degrees of immunity to these new bacterial forms. These spirochetal bacteria spread rapidly throughout the industrialized world and caused Vincent's disease. Most likely, the reason for this was because treatment methods were inadequate; therefore, it was impossible to eliminate the bacteria from infected patients completely, which in turn facilitated its spread throughout the world. Despite the peoples' immune systems mounting an attack against the disease, it is likely that some bacteria survived and became indigenous to those exposed to the bacteria. These bacteria were then transmitted from parents to children, generation after generation, until the present day. Evidence suggests that people did build varying degrees of immunity to the disease. Treponema Vincenti, a spirochete that was introduced so many years ago, can be isolated in mouths of people today. Whether it is this spirochete specifically that causes systemic disease, similar spirochetes, or mutations of these spirochetes, remains to be discovered.

Later in the book, I will present examples of periodontal disease and peri-implant infections caused by these indigenous bacteria. Many implants have been lost because of an infection that either was introduced into the oral environment many years ago or has recently been transmitted to humans via other vectors.

Chapter 4
Important Clues Learned from Other Spirochetal Diseases and Correlating These to the Relationship between Periodontal and Heart Disease

Once I returned from Cabo San Lucas with my first rough draft of this book, I decided to study other spirochetal diseases. One of these was syphilis, which was disseminated throughout the indigenous population of the Americas when the Europeans first discovered the continents. Europeans interacted and bred with local populations, which didn't have any resistance to the disease. It is important to note that the bacteria that cause Vincent's disease, Treponema Vincenti, are spirochetes similar to those that cause syphilis, Treponema Pallidum (both from the genus Treponema). I also studied Lyme disease, a spirochetal illness caused by the bacteria Borrelia burgdorferi. Since the lifecycle of syphilis was discovered and described at the turn of the 19th century, and since today we also have a more complete understanding of the lifecycle of Borrelia burgdorferi, is it possible that these three illnesses, being spirochetal in nature, share more than just a few traits in common?

Syphilis is a venereal disease that is usually transmitted during sexual intercourse by someone who has an active infection. The spirochete that causes syphilis is thought to have the ability to penetrate the mucus membrane of the urethra (lining of the penis), the vaginal lining, the skin of the penis as well as any other skin, including oral mucosa, with which it comes into contact. Once it gains access to the underlying tissue, it incubates for a period of ten to forty days and then forms a painless boil or lesion on the skin called a chancre. The nearby lymph nodes become swollen and hard. After a period of time, this lesion heals without scarring.

The fact that syphilis spirochetes can penetrate the skin of a penis or the vaginal mucosa suggests that other spirochetes, including oral spirochetes, might be able to penetrate cell membranes or tissue easily. This book provides an example in chapter five of a spirochete penetrating a mucosal cell located in the gingival sulcus. Thus, it is not far-fetched to presume that a spirochete can penetrate the endothelial lining of blood vessels and cause atherosclerotic lesions. It is well known that oral bacteria enter the bloodstream from gum-diseased tissue, and that spirochetes have been seen in the blood. These oral spirochetes gain access to the bloodstream via bacteremias, which are caused by manipulation of the infected gums of patients with periodontal disease. Bacteremias can result from any or all of the following activities: chewing food, normal teeth brushing and flossing, prophylactic teeth cleaning at the dentist's office, probing of the pockets of gums by dentists or by any manipulation of the diseased gum tissue. As the book proceeds, it will become evident that diseased gums are not a good condition to have.

In syphilis, if the primary lesion is not recognized and treated with antibiotics, then the disease goes into the secondary stage about six weeks later. The secondary stage is characterized by fever, copper-hued and multiple skin eruptions all over the body with no itching, severe pain in the joints and the periosteum (tissue that covers the bone). If this stage is not treated, then the disease goes into a dormant or resting phase. This dormant latent phase can last for years.

When the immune system becomes compromised later in life, syphilis enters a tertiary stage, the most dangerous stage of the disease. This later stage is characterized by a set of peculiar skin affections, including scabby boils, gumma, which can occur anywhere in the body, and successive crops of bubbles, which eventually dissipate, leaving dark spots on the skin. It is associated with multiple mental disorders. It is also associated with the same bone abscess types of lesions that are found in advanced periodontal and Lyme disease. The symptoms found in the third phase of syphilis are similar to those of Vincent's disease and traditional periodontal disease. Even though these two spirochetes, Vincent's disease and syphilis, are not exactly the same genetically, they come from the same genus category, Treponema, and look very much alike under the microscope. There may be differences, but it is possible they have similar survival strategies and lifecycles.

In the old literature (1907)[27], I found illustrations that show various forms of the syphilis spirochete. It has a typical "corkscrew" shape, which seems to be its active form (figure 3, next page). As it transitions before its death to a reproductive stage, it forms granules inside its cell body. When the cell membrane breaks down, the granules are dispersed into the body fluid for later regeneration into their viable active spirochete form. Later, in 1912[28], Hindle shows emergence of a granular "coccoid" form of spirochetes (figure 4 and 5). It was reported back then that these protective forms are resistant to traditional antibiotic treatment. Once the spirochetes transform and retreat into the

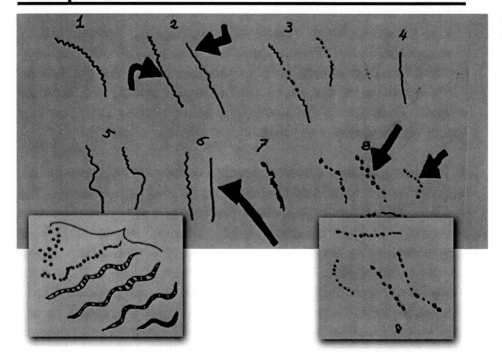

FIGURES 3 (top), 4 (bottom left), and 5 (bottom right). Fg. 3: Live forms of T. Pallidum, Bull Soc. Med. Hsp. Paris Vol. 24:114-116, 1907. Fg. 4: Cocco-id bodies in blood. Hindel, 1912, Emergence of granular "coccoid" forms from spirochetes. Fg 5: Year 1907, Paris, France, Jacquet and Sezary line drawings of syphilis granular "constellation" forms of T. pallidum.

body's tissue in the granular or cystic form, they live in relative harmony with the body until the immunity of the host is compromised or diminished. Later in the book, I theorize how inflammation is the most likely stimulus that triggers the bacteria's transformation into a viable "corkscrew"-causing form of disease.

A recent resurgence of syphilis in modern society demonstrates that penicillin does not effectively eliminate the disease. Thus, new methods are needed to diagnose syphilis and to monitor the success or failure of therapies. It is now known that unless the disease is diagnosed and treated early, it is impossible to eradicate the pathogen that causes it. Recognition of the aberrant forms of this pathogen is pertinent for diagnosing the sensitivity of the treatment modality used in the various stages of the infection[29].

A study of Lyme disease, another spirochetal disease, is also sobering. This disease causes similar problems to those of syphilis and is linked to heart disease, multiple neurological diseases, premature birth, spontaneous abortions, arthritis, and is related to many other inflammatory diseases. Pam Weintraub, in her book *Cure Unknown*[30], details the discovery, the history of treatment, and the devastating chronic debilitating symptoms produced by Lyme disease. This book is probably the best source for information on the research, controversy, and long-term treatment of Lyme disease. The medical community is deeply divided regarding the treatment of Lyme disease. Evidently, this disease is very persistent and is not always cured by an initial treatment. It has a secondary phase that is similar to syphilis in its symptomology and the organism's lifecycle. No single antibiotic or combination of antibiotics appears to be capable of completely eradicating the infection, and treatment failures or relapses are reported with all current regimens, although they are less frequent with early, aggressive treatment[31]. This is one more spirochete that seems to present secondary complications to the sufferer if it is allowed to disseminate throughout the body via the bloodstream and cause problems[32].

Recent compelling evidence by MacDonald[33] illustrates that the Lyme disease spirochete, Borrelia burgdorferi, has granular and cystic forms that are distinct from one other. Using DNA markers, MacDonald was able to find cysts in Alzheimer's plaques containing the spirochete's DNA. He feels that the plaques originate from cysts of the Borrelia burgdorferi spirochete that cause Lyme disease (figures 6–11). Up until now, the spirochetes from syphilis and Lyme disease have been shown to have similar to identical forms, including granules, cysts, and other irregular

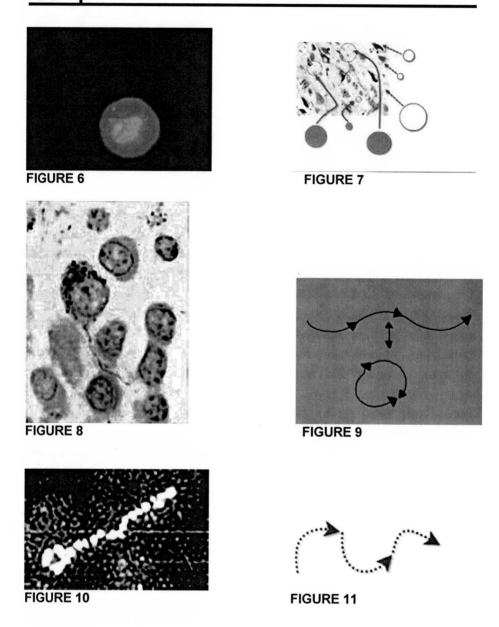

FIGURE 6

FIGURE 7

FIGURE 8

FIGURE 9

FIGURE 10

FIGURE 11

forms besides the typical spiral. In chapter five, I will describe how all oral spirochetes have the same morphological forms.

Figures 6-11:

Figure 6 is a photograph showing the cystic form of Borrelia burgdorferi (Lyme disease spirochete) from spinal fluid culture, Magnification 1000x.

Figure 7 shows the cyst insertion into brain sites.

Figure 8 shows granular bodies within the hippocampus nerve in Alzheimer's disease. Original slide was taken from Harvard McLean Brain bank. This case was used in Reference 8 (Polymerase Chain Reaction - Molecular Interogation for Flagellin B DNA study), 1000x magnification.

Figure 9 is a schematic line drawing of corkscrew to cyst conversion of Borrelia burgdorferi (Lyme disease spirochete).

Figure 10 shows Borrelia burgdorferi (Lyme disease spirochete) with murine monoclonal antibiotic H5332 fingerprint from fresh brain Alzheimer's disease, in the year 1987. The photograph shows the presence of spirochete granular bodies in Alzheimer's lesions.

Figure 11 is a line drawing that illustrates the segmentation of a spirochete into coccoid bodies. Each coccoid granule contains DNA for reproduction of a spirochete.

I also discussed DNA markers in a personal conversation with MacDonald[34]. Specifically, I asked him whether the DNA markers used in his work represented the Borrelia burgdorferi spirochete itself or other spirochetes in general. If Lyme disease were the cause of Alzheimer's disease, then Alzheimer's would be more prevalent in areas of the world where deer tick populations are greater. However, Alzheimer's disease is evenly spread throughout the population. I believe—and MacDonald concurred—that it is more likely that oral spirochetes also could cause the plaques he observed, since periodontal disease is evenly distributed throughout the population. Some months after this conversation, I examined atherosclerosis plaques provided to me by a researcher studying atherosclerotic plaques located in the aorta. During this examination in my laboratory, I found morphological spore-like forms identical to those that I have found in periodontal disease. To date, little is known about spores—especially those formed from oral spirochetes—but such a discovery definitively links oral spirochetes with atherosclerotic heart disease. The chronological process of my discovery of these bodies, both in the gingival sulcus and the aorta, will be presented in chapter five. The clues MacDonald found while researching the cause of Lyme disease may have inadvertently resulted in my discovery of the causative agent for not only plaque-forming neurological diseases, including Alzheimer's disease, but also for heart disease.

Lyme disease is transmitted initially from the white-footed mouse via tick to the white-tailed deer, or visa-versa, via the deer tick. Its primary reservoir invertebrate is the deer tick and the primate reservoir is the white-footed mouse and/or the white-tailed deer. The spirochete is transmitted to humans via the deer tick. Dairy cattle and other food animals can also be infected with the Lyme disease spirochete. The pathogen may also be transmitted orally to laboratory animals, without the deer tick. Therefore, the possibility exists that Lyme disease is a food contaminant and can be transmitted via ingestion of spirochetal spore-infested food.[35]

An investigative reporter, Bryan Rosner in his book *The Top 10 Lyme Disease Treatments*[36], reports research that the Lyme disease organism exists in three distinct forms: an active spirochete, a cell-wall-deficient (CWD) form and a cystic form. The active form is very mobile, spiral/drill-like, and is capable of penetrating dense tissue directly and bone via blood capillaries. It can infect intracellular tissue and converts rapidly into a cell-wall-deficient and/or cyst form when threatened. The cell-wall deficient form lacks a cell wall, which makes targeting it with antibiotics and/or the body's immune system much more difficult. It is also capable of infecting the insides of cells, and of converting Vitamin D to an immunosuppressive hormone known a 1,25-D. It also causes auto-immunity and clumps together in dense colonies (with the inner layer of spirochetes in either active, "cell-wall-deficient" or cyst forms where they are un-reachable by antibiotics and the immune system).

The cyst form of Borrelia is dormant, immobile, and does not cause symptoms. It can survive antibiotics, starvation, pH changes, hydrogen peroxide, temperature variations, and most other adverse conditions. It converts back to the spirochete form when conditions are more favorable.

There is evidence that oral spirochetes are similar to those found in syphilis and Lyme disease and that these can move from the initial lesion to distal locations. Smithe and Riviere[37] found evidence of oral Treponema in the brains of Alzheimer's disease patients. Miklossy[38] observed spirochetes in the blood of those with Alzheimer's disease. These facts provide additional evidence that spirochetes in general may cause or contribute to plaque-forming neurological diseases.

The study of tertiary syphilis and chronic Lyme disease show that each can produce similar debilitating long-term diseases. Both diseases produce heart disease and mental problems, including short- and long-term memory loss, dementia, schizophrenia, arthritis, autoimmune, and many other chronic diseases. Lyme disease is called the "stealth disease" because it mimics many other chronic diseases. In chapter eight, in the discussion of Multiple Missing Tooth Syndrome, I will demonstrate how pa-tients with periodontal disease, presumably related to oral spirochetes, produce the same, but a subtler, slow-developing and a more chronic form of the same type of diseases as Lyme disease and syphilis. In oral spirochetosis, the acute phase is various degrees of inflammation and disease of the "gums." Later stages take a lifetime to develop into systemic chronic inflammatory diseases that catch up with people at later more vulnerable years.

Another spirochete that is thought to populate the gingival sulcus is Helicobacter pylori[39], which is the bacteria that causes stomach ulcers and cancer. This bacterium, like Borrelia burgdorferi (Lyme disease) or mutations of Borrelia, is also capable of transforming to coccoid (cystoid) forms and then reversing back to normal mobile forms[40]. This spirochete has been discovered, forgotten and rediscovered at least three times in the past one hundred years. The literature supports the fact that these pylori spirochetes also develop resistance to antibiotics. A more thorough study of pylori would probably demonstrate that it has some of the same characteristics as syphilis and Lyme disease. One thing is for certain: Pylori have been linked to stomach cancer.

A long list of research papers also report granular, cysts, and other forms to spirochetes[41]. Intense research needs to be directed toward understanding and treating oral spirochetal infections that seem very similar to their spirochetal cousins.

The more I study "spirochetosis," the more I am convinced that if you study one type of spirochete, then you can understand all of them. Therefore, by studying syphilis, Lyme disease, pylori, and the other spirochetal diseases, you will find they are all similar to each other and their survival strategies are strikingly similar. Some experts with whom I have consulted agree there are no good spirochetes. All other spirochetal infections in the body, excluding oral spirochetes, are taken seriously by physicians and aggressively treated. Why haven't dentists taken oral spirochetes more seriously?

Most people have these oral spirochetes bacteria without any signs or symptoms. The bacteria are passed from mother to child; hence, what once appeared to be a genetic disease now appears to be a communicable and/or food-borne disease. Over the years, it appears people have developed greater immunity to these oral spirochetes. However, when the immune system is compromised, the conditions become ripe for transformation and reemergence of disease. These once thought as only locally invasive indigenous oral spirochetes in the gingival sulcus can become virulent and not only cause active periodontal disease but also systemic manifestation of oral spirochetosis. Conditions such as diabetes (with its friable blood vessels), low-level scurvy (poor nutrition, especially insufficient vitamin C[42]) that results in blood vessel breakdown, or any other disease that results in a lowering of immune system function, such as dental infections, can cause this phenomenon. What is especially true is that it is possible for spirochetal forms to reactivate in the endothelial lining of arteries in the heart, causing a final inflammatory response that results in a heart attack. In blood vessels, it is postulated that an activation of the spores can produce blood clots.

Is it possible that atherosclerotic heart disease is related to, or is the final manifestation of oral spirochetosis, similar to the tertiary stage of syphilis? Let us examine the evidence. The literature, as mentioned earlier, shows that Vincent's disease is highly contagious. Also, the research I have done on patients in my clinic using a microscope, indicates that oral spirochetes are easy to transmit. Spirochetes in families where no intimate contact is practiced between mother and children are yet found to be identical. The transmission of oral spirochetes is difficult to understand without a spore transmission theory. Do we really understand the method of transmission? Oral spirochetes are anaerobic and hence do not tolerate oxygen well. The literature I found describes how difficult it is for these spirochetes to disseminate in experimental conditions. Most are not even culturable in the laboratory. Therefore, as I started this investigation, I wondered why these bacteria are so easy to transmit from person to person. Maybe they are also transmitted via food-borne vectors, but how?

My research included gathering as many of the old textbooks on bacteriology as possible, in order that I might find this transmission mode. I found only one reference on oral spirochete spores or granules, dated 1960. It stated, *"External granules may become free from the cell and in old cultures, containing granular forms when examined by dark-field microscopy, have been shown to give rise to typical spirochetes on subculture to fresh medium-the granules may therefore be a stage in the lifecycle of the organism[43]."* These granules appeared on the surface of the spirochetes just prior to their death. The bacteriologist who reported this finding also observed these spores developing into duplicate multiple spirochetes.

In more recent literature, Wolf et al[44] reported quasi (different)-multi-cellular-bodies of Treponema denticola, the most common oral spirochete. They analyzed its forms using electron microscope methods and found it had four forms: normal helical, twisted spirochetes that formed plaits, twisted spirochetes that formed club-like structures, and spherical bodies of different sizes. The researchers theorized that such forms were better able to resist adverse conditions such as antibiotics and toxins. (See drawings of the various forms in figure 12, next page).

In 1999, De Ciccio et al[45] reported finding morphological variations of the same oral spirochete, Treponema denticola, in the form of spherical bodies. Up until this time in history, it was not known what influenced oral spirochetes to form these bodies. The authors of this report attributed the changes to environmen-

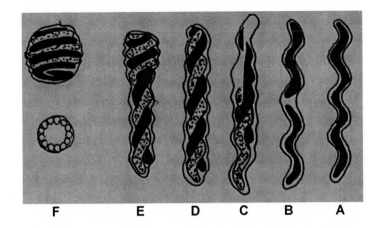

Figure 12: Schematic drawings that illustrate the transformation of Treponema Denticola (oral gum disease spirochete) from the helical form to the spore "spherical body" form. (Note: Order is from right to left).

  a. Typical helical form of Treponema starting from the monoforme spirochete.
  b. Separation of the protoplasmic cylinders of dividing Treponemas, outer sheath remains intact.
  c. Movement of the two Treponemas in contrary directions initiates plait formation.
  d. Plait form as an intermediate form toward a spherical body
  e. Further movements compress the individual Treponemas to a club form.
  f. Final stage: the spherical body form containing several Treponemas: the upper picture depicts the cross-section.

tal stress and related their findings to periodontal disease by stating that the "spherical bodies" represent resting forms of the organisms. Their presence corresponds with periods of disease quiescence or non-activity. In my studies I have examined the plaque taken from patients with no evidence of periodontal disease using the microscope and found the active helical form of spirochetes, but no periodontal disease. Unknown to me for years, but after finding literature references to these spore forms, I went back and studied the videos of these examinations. I found the inactive forms and spore-like forms, as well. The chronology of this discovery will be discussed later in the book.

Even though this transitional phenomenon is not commonly known in clinical dentistry, it is logical to conclude that friable bacteria, which are sensitive to oxygen and resistant to transmission from one experimental subject to another, are able to produce a spore that is easily transmitted within populations. How is it possible for syphilis-causing spirochetes to live in the body for so many years without the body's defense mechanisms destroying them? The answer is that the body's immune system, toxins and antibiotics cannot destroy cysts, spores, spherical bodies, cell-wall-deficient-forms, and/or the granules that spirochetes form to survive. I mention all the diverse forms because different authors use different descriptions to describe what might be the same entity.

Now that I have shown the similarities between the various spirochetal diseases found in the medical literature, I will continue to describe the chronological sequence of discovery I experienced over the last year and a half. Now armed with the knowledge of other spirochetal forms and the scant literature (three references) of the same oral spirochete (Treponema denticola) forms, I eventually discovered the same altered spirochetal forms in my own periodontal disease patients. And then, to my delight, I found these bodies in the atherosclerotic plaque lesions of the aorta.

Chapter 5
Oral Spirochetosis Associated with Dental Implants; Important Clues to Systemic Disease

Evidence indicates that all spirochetes, including syphilis and Lyme disease, have similar, if not identical, survival strategies. Most dental clinicians do not understand this. If they did, and they knew that such spirochetes are present in periodontal disease, then they would be trained to recognize the conditions they cause. Microscopes would be present in every dental office that treats periodontal disease. Obviously, dentists do not have the ability to diagnose spirochetal illness or use microscopes, but it remains extremely important that they understand the bacteria they are treating.

Once I understood spores (spherical bodies and cysts) as well as other forms of spirochetes, I immediately had a better understanding of periodontal disease and, particularly, at what stage it was present in my patients' mouths. Prior to my knowledge about spirochetes and for seven years, I had been diagnosing gum disease with a microscope, but knew nothing about spores. After discovering this phenomenon, I questioned dental microbiology colleagues to discover whether anyone else knew anything about them, but it turns out no one did.

Syphilis spores or granules were once recognized and understood more than one hundred years ago, but evidently, this understanding was lost in the vast old archives of medical and dental literature. I have asked some of my physician friends if they knew about these bodies. Specifically, they did not. Most were under the impression that syphilis is easily treated with penicillin and that was all there was to it. It was obvious to me that little information is known about the survival strategy of syphilis spirochetes. Even the existence of chronic Lyme disease is in dispute. It is little wonder then, that dentists have no knowledge of these altered spirochetal entities. When I was alerted to the fact that spore forms of spirochetes exist, I surmised I would find them in dental plaque. And, in fact, I did, in every single microscopic examination of periodontal disease I performed. Over the years, I performed electronic recordings of the microscope sessions I had with my patients, in order to document and track treatment success. When I went back and reviewed their electronic records, I found that such spores were everywhere, and were especially prevalent after antibiotic treatment.

Prior to my knowledge about spirochetal spores, I had observed these floating dark granular bodies in plaque samples that were taken after antibiotic treatment but, at the time, hadn't recognized what they were. Patients would even ask me, "What is all that dirt floating around under the microscope?" I would tell them I didn't know, but that I thought it was dead bacteria. Later, upon reexaminations of the post-antibiotic samples, I realized the material was not dirt, but rather, spirochetes that had been induced into spore form by the antibiotics, but not eradicated. They had been in the microscopic field for years, but I had never recognized them for what they were.

Clinical Cases that Led to the Discovery of the Role of Spirochetes and Spores in Implant Dentistry Failures

In my role as an implant dentist, I have come across numerous clinical cases over the last twenty years that implicate spirochetes in the bone loss that results from oral implant failures. In the next section, I will present cases that were truly remarkable once understood because they demonstrate the similarity of oral spirochetes to other spirochetal diseases. These are the cases I spent the most time writing about during the first week of my vacation in Cabo San Lucas. I didn't know during that first week that these cases would be part of this book. However, that is the way this whole project has gone, with unexpected surprises. I would theorize something, research it and then find evidence for that theory. Whenever I needed more collaboration, the right researcher would show up at just the right time, and each new discovery would lead to another, until all the details of my theory would eventually fall into place.

These next cases are a few representative examples of patients I've treated. Their cases illustrate the connection between spirochetes, periodontal disease and implant failures. From these cases, I have learned I must treat spirochetal infection before implant treatment can commence. After that, it is the patient's responsibility to follow up their periodontal disease treatment with daily home care to prevent spores from reemerging to cause further disease or implant failure. Spirochetal infections are destructive to dental implants because they cause severe bone loss around the implants as well as acute infection and inflammation. The fact that such destructive infections can cause bone loss around dental implants that is typically seen in other spirochetal infestations, including syphilis and Lyme disease, provides one more piece of evidence that they may also be virulent enough to be related to other systemic diseases such as heart disease. Also, data from these cases proves that antibiotics do not eliminate oral spirochetes, as in other spirochetal diseases; they only force them into a more protected spore form.

More detailed descriptions of the following cases can be found in Appendix II for those interested in more in-depth clinical information regarding the cases.

CASE #1

A thirty-seven-year-old woman of Vietnamese descent needed three implants to replace a missing molar and bicuspid tooth. Within months after the implants were completed, bone loss occurred around the top of her dental implants. I determined, with the aid of my microscope, that the bone loss was caused by a spirochetal infection (figure 16).

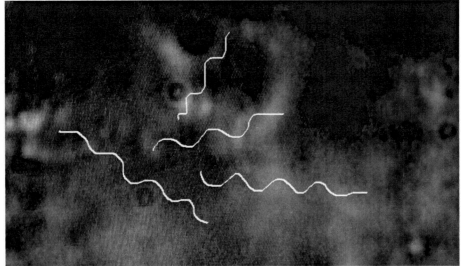

Figure 16: Graphically enhanced spirochetes that are very difficult to visualize when not in motion. The white forms are spirochetes in stop motion.

At the onset of and during treatment, the patient never exhibited any traditional signs or symptoms of periodontal disease. I observed that the patient had excellent oral hygiene. After discovering the spirochetal infection, the patient was treated systemically with antibiotics for two weeks. During the second week, while the patient was still on antibiotics, I performed another microscopic examination, cleaned her teeth and performed corrective surgery on her implants. This microscopic examination was done prior to my knowledge about the existence of spirochetal spores. Before I finish my observations about this patient, I want to describe the other patients who were treated sequentially after her. At this microscopic and DVD electronic recording exam I hadn't discovered spores yet.

CASE #2

A fifty-four-year-old man with periodontal disease had his upper teeth extracted and a custom implant placed. Over the next twelve years, episodes of infection would occur around the upper implant, and these were treated with various antibiotics; however, the infections always returned. During those years, and without the aid of a microscope, I did not know whether the patient was getting re-infected from some outside source, or whether indigenous bacteria were causing the infections. In 2007, I performed microscopic bacterial studies on his plaque and infected tissue. The results revealed a spirochete infection. I placed the patient on antibiotics, and we scheduled a visit for the implant to be removed. At the end of the two weeks, the patient requested, if it would be at all possible, to save the implant.

I then performed another examination on his dental plaque using a microscope two weeks into his antibiotic treatment and concluded that the antibiotic regimen had not been adequate for killing the spirochetes, because the bacteria had somehow developed resistance to the drugs over the years. The implant was then removed.

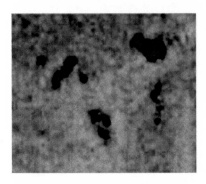

Figure 23: After antibiotic treatment, you can observe a viable spirochete that survived the antibiotics, as well as adjacent granular forms.

This was the first periodontal disease case that I had following my discovery of spores from other spirochetes, i.e., syphilis and Lyme disease, and which provided me with the opportunity to find spores in periodontal disease. I was elated when, in fact, a microscopic study of his plaque revealed a field that was filled with what I assumed to be multiple spores, spherical bodies and/or granular forms. These altered forms were found in the sample I had taken from the gingival sulcus after over more than one week of antibiotic treatment (figure 23). They appeared as dense granular doughnut-shaped substances surrounded by a white halo, with a hollow light refractive center. Such forms were identical to other spirochete spore forms described in the medical literature. Needless to say, I was thrilled about this discovery, because it was evidence that oral spirochetes are similar in form to other types of spirochetes. Also, the spirochetes I saw in this patient must have had the ability to convert to different forms (as evidenced by the presence of the spores), thus reflecting a survival strategy that is found in other spirochetes.

CASE #3

A forty-three-year-old woman came into my office for an implant treatment. I extracted several of her teeth and placed implants in 2001, and periodically examined her over the next several years. At her most recent follow-up examination, I discovered severe bone loss on one natural tooth adjacent to bone loss on an implant. I also observed seven to eight millimeters of bone loss from two other adjacent implants. When I examined her plaque and infected tissue with my microscope, I found a spirochetal infection. I once again placed her on antibiotics, and after a week, while she was still on antibiotics, I removed the single infected tooth and adjacent implant. I also microscopically examined the granulation tissue (infected tissue) from around the two other implants and found it was loaded with spirochetal spores throughout (figure 28). The large clump of material contained many spirochetes radiating concentrically from its surface—as in, spilling out from a center. I concluded that spirochetes were the reason for the implant failure. Again, as in the previous case, I found similar spherical, spore-like forms (figures 29–30).

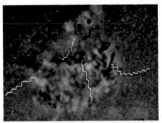

Figure 28: Infected tissue that was removed from the bottom of a periodontal pocket adjacent to a failing implant. Notice the large granular structure with highlighted spirochetes radiating from the outside surface.

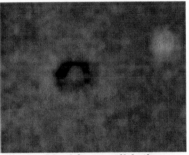

Figure 29: After antibiotic treatment, granular forms were found with a white colored halo, a dark colored grainy appearing layer and a hollow center.

CASE #4

A forty-five-year-old woman came to my office with periodontal disease. Her condition

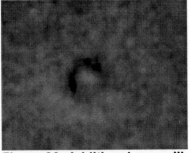

Figure 30: Additional spore-like formations.

required a tooth extraction and an implant placement. This patient had a history of five failed periodontal surgeries over the past twenty years. I examined her dental plaque under the microscope before treating her with antibiotics and discovered a severe spirochete infection, just as I had with the patients in the

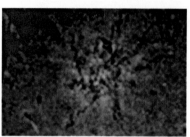

Figure 33: a cystic form with hundreds of granules inside, and large spirochetes radiating from it.

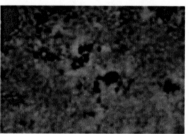

Figure 34: granular bodies formed after antibiotic treatment, presumably from the protected form of the spirochetes. Notice white halo with ring of black granular substance and a white hollow center.

previous two cases. Large ball-shaped clumps filled with an unknown granular-appearing material with hundreds of spirochetes attached to the outside wall and radiating concentrically from the surface were observed (figure 33). I placed her on antibiotics and reexamined her tissue under the microscope a week later, while she was still on the antibiotics. I observed that the granule-filled forms (figure 34) were still present; however, I did not find any active spirochetes. As in the previous cases, there were numerous spore-like forms with the same white halo around them with a hollow light refractive center and dense, grainy-appearing material in the form of a flat-donut shaped body. The central light refractive material looks like a flashlight shining out from the center of the spore when observed with a phase contrast microscope. I cannot help but think the spirochete can in some way communicate with me using this flashlight. It seems to be saying to me, "Here I am, what are you going to do about it?"

Medical literature has proven that periodontal disease is related to bone loss and can cause implant failures.[46] [47] [48] In case No. 1, however, I found no clinical evidence of periodontal disease. Studies have shown that those who initially show no traditional signs or symptoms of periodontal disease often have, in their gingival sulci, the bacteria that cause it, especially the spirochetes. Generally speaking, the literature identifies two types of spirochetes; the first produces disease, and the second are non-pathogenic, or non-disease producing. Patients with disease-producing spirochetes are three times more likely to develop periodontitis within a year than those healthy patients who have the non-virulent type of spirochete. The pathogenic-related spirochetes are the ones that are most likely to cause infection[49]. Unfortunately, in the clinical practice of implant dentistry, it is impossible to differentiate between the two groups of spirochetes. Based on my many years of microscopic examination of infections associated with failing implants, I have observed many morphologic types of spirochetes in diseased tissue. The jury is still out, in my opinion, as to which of these two types of spirochetes, if not both, can cause implant failures. In my research, and in general, spirochetes seem to be a "marker bacteria" for periodontal infections that cause bone loss and implant failure.

The Vietnamese woman mentioned in case No. 1 provides an example of a patient who had spirochetal bacteria but no initial clinical signs of periodontal disease. However, within a few months after placing her implants, I observed infection and swelling around the necks of the implants. In addition, X-rays showed bone loss around the implants, and a study using the microscope revealed an active infection teeming with predominately small, but very active, spirochetes.

Since this patient did not have any initial signs or symptoms of periodontal disease, I did not complete any of the routine microscopic bacterial studies that are normally done on patients with gum disease. However, upon discovery of the bacteria (predominately spirochetes) associated with the bone loss in her mouth, I performed a microscopic examination, after the fact, of the gingival sulci in other areas of her mouth. Not surprisingly, the same microbiological pattern of spirochetal bacteria was observed in these areas. Even though medical literature reports these bacteria can be present in healthy appearing gum sulci without any signs or symptoms of periodontal disease, knowledge of this fact eludes implant dentists. It is impossible to recognize this pre-disease process before an implant is placed, unless microscopic evaluations are done on every patient. This adds yet one more complication to the already challenging field of implant dentistry, because it means that dentists who place dental implants must now also become proficient in bacteriology and examine every patient for spirochetes before any implant dentistry can be performed.

However, microscopic examination of plaque samples taken from the gingival sulci is the only effective method of diagnosis I am aware of; therefore, dentists must have microscopes and know how to use them to make accurate diagnoses. Other tests, such as DNA and BANA, test for only a few of the 57 known species of oral spirochetes, while the microscope detects all of the spirochetes, as well as their organization with other bacteria.

Morphologically Identical Spore-like Forms Discovered in the Atherosclerotic Lesions of Blood Vessels

After finding what looked like spores in the periodontal lesions of the aforementioned patients, it became obvious to me that there must be identical spores in the atherosclerotic plaques of their blood vessels. However, because it is impossible to access these patients' blood vessels, in order to solve the last piece of the puzzle, I realized I had to find another way to make the connection.

Coincidentally, a new patient who would be instrumental in proving the last step of the periodontal-heart disease equation arrived at my office for implant dentistry in October 2007. This patient, named Corbett, was a researcher, and during our first visit, he informed me he had once sold an orthopedic company. This fact was ironic to me, because I am also involved in this industry. I manufacture custom endosteal implants, an orthopedic appliance for tooth replacement in patients with severe bone loss; that is, people who have very little bone in their jaws for traditional root-form (screw-type) implants. We discussed our mutual experiences together, and I then told him I was studying oral bacteria that cause problems with implants and natural teeth. I also mentioned I thought these bacteria were related to heart disease.

Corbett told me he and his biotech company had been investigating atherosclerotic lesions for more than ten years at different universities, including the University of California, San Diego. I could not believe what I was hearing. My next comment to him was that I needed to see a histological slide of an atherosclerotic lesion in the worst way. The expression on his face when I told him about the spores was remarkable, but he didn't divulge to me at that moment why he had such an expression of amazement. It took two more appointments with him before I gained his trust (since he said his research material was top secret) and he revealed to me the reason for his expression. He had seen these same bodies in his studies of atherosclerotic plaque, but didn't know what they were. He finally agreed to let me see the slides with the fresh atherosclerotic lesions. It was a Monday night in November and the week that I would be lecturing on the subject of oral spirochetosis at the American Academy of Implant

Dentistry (AAID) in Las Vegas. Needless to say, I was very excited, because I had been given the slides for one night. I was excited because I had hoped to obtain new information from the slides, which I could then present at the lecture.

Corbett delivered to me a large case of histology slides, most representing cases of atherosclerosis that had already been treated by his company's "secret" technique. Hence, these were of no value to me. There were, however, several slides of fresh plaques containing various atherosclerotic lesions. Immediately, and nervously, I placed the first slide into my microscope and focused it to a magnification of 1000x. After only a few seconds, I identified spores identical to those found in periodontal lesions. These spores had unique morphologic characteristics that were unmistakable; the familiar dark-colored, granular, doughnut-shaped body with a light-refractive material center, surrounded by a faint halo (figures 35–41, next two pages). This shape precisely mirrors the morphology of the spores found in periodontal lesions. I digitally recorded movies of the samples and prepared them to be shown at the AAID meeting that week. It took three weeks for me to come down off of the discovery-high that I experienced as a result of what I learned from these slides.

Subsequently, the next question I asked myself was, What possible benefit would there be for spirochetes to find their way into the circulatory system and then into the endothelial lining of blood vessels, where they produce spores? The answer to this question must relate to some strategy that the spirochetes use in their lifecycle for survival. Then, it occurred to me that blood vessels are also located everywhere in the body, including the muscles (or meat). Meat ensures spirochetes' survival because they are then passed on and disseminated to other animals when the host's meat is consumed.

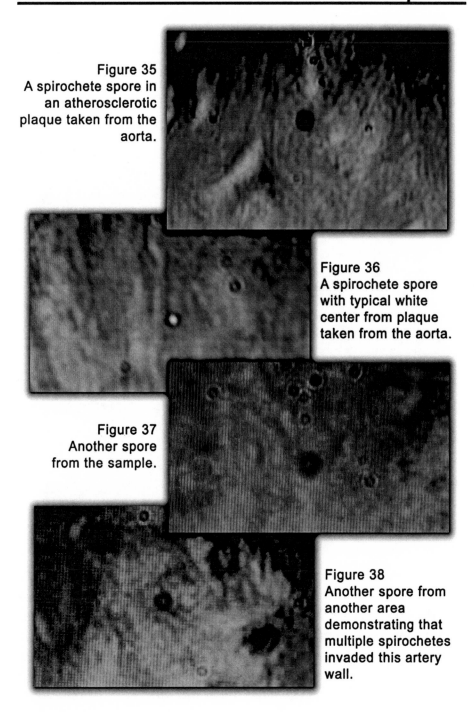

Figure 35
A spirochete spore in an atherosclerotic plaque taken from the aorta.

Figure 36
A spirochete spore with typical white center from plaque taken from the aorta.

Figure 37
Another spore from the sample.

Figure 38
Another spore from another area demonstrating that multiple spirochetes invaded this artery wall.

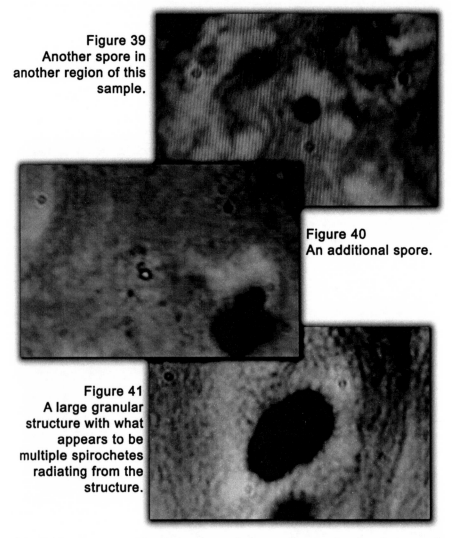

Figure 39
Another spore in
another region of this
sample.

Figure 40
An additional spore.

Figure 41
A large granular
structure with what
appears to be
multiple spirochetes
radiating from the
structure.

The idea that muscle is meat and that meat is the food that other animals eat, including humans, prompted me to investigate whether there is a food-borne vector that we have not considered and that is responsible for spirochete transmission in humans. It was mentioned earlier that Lyme disease can be spread to other animals by consuming contaminated meat[50]. Why then shouldn't it be possible for all spirochetes, including oral spirochetes, to be disseminated to other animals through the consumption of meat where spirochetal spores reside? I surmised that this additional transmission vector must exist in order to ensure the spirochete's survival. I went to Medline to research the idea. I used the words, "spirochetes" and "cattle" in my search. To my amazement, the veterinary research literature revealed that similar spirochetes have been found in cattle. Furthermore, spirochetes that are similar to the oral spirochetes found in humans (bearing a 95 percent similarity to Treponema denticola and 98 percent similarity Treponema Vincenti) cause digital dermatitis (an ulcerative condition) affecting the feet of cows and sheep.[51] [52] [53] [54]

The spirochetes in cattle are not only found in dermatitis lesions, but, as has been demonstrated from this book and other literature, it is the nature of a spirochete to distribute itself throughout the circulatory system to all parts of the body, including the meat. It is beyond coincidence that the two very similar spirochetes found in cattle and sheep also cause periodontal disease and Vincent's disease, respectively, in humans. Furthermore, I theorize that it is the Vincent's disease spirochete, Treponema vincenti, which started the whole atherosclerotic disease epidemic in the first place, beginning in the early 1900s. Since similar, if not identical, spirochetes are found in cattle, it is likely that these spirochetes in their protected spore form serve as food-borne vectors of transmission to humans. It is hard to understand how the highly contagious disease, Trench mouth, was spread throughout the industrialized world so rapidly by what was thought to be oral transmission. Due to the evidence that we have found, it is much more likely that it was spread through food contamination. Either way, whether it spread orally or via contaminated food, it is vital that dentists diagnose and treat any new spirochetal infestation in the gingival sulcus.

Hamburger is notoriously bacteria-laden. When pour-plate (a type of culture medium) cultures of hamburger are examined microscopically for 18 hours at room temperature, micro-colonies of "cell-wall-deficient" or spore forms of spirochetal bacteria are found to be prevalent. However, it is evident that these forms are not recognized as spirochetes and are usually identified as "normal flora" overgrowth[55].

Dr. Richard J. Fink, a pioneer in the study of inflammatory atherosclerosis, believes that an unknown injurious agent is involved in the disease process. This agent causes the inflamma-tory immune cell, which is meant to heal disease, to turn on itself and thereby cause inflammatory atherosclerotic heart disease. Since I found what appeared to be spirochetal spores in the atherosclerotic plaque, I wondered if these spores had something to do with this inflammatory response. What happens to the inflammatory cells to transform them into something that is not recognized by the immune system as friendly? It seems evident after reading Fink's book that the leucocytes, primarily mono-cytes (inflammatory cells), are the first to show up to defend the body against the injurious agent. These then undergo transfor-mation into macrophages (another type of immune cell) and eventually become fatty streaks that populate the atherosclerotic plaque. According to Ellen, quoted in the first chapter, spiro-chetes have the ability to evade the immune system. Because of this, it can be postulated that spirochetes are involved in in-flammatory atherosclerotic disease and have something to do with the infamous injurious agent. The evidence of spore-like bodies in the atherosclerotic plaque indicated that spirochetal DNA or cyst-forms have evaded the immune system and are potentially active in the plaque, causing an inflammatory reac-tion. A short video clip from MacDonald's research illustrates a lymphocyte engulfing a spirochete (photos of which are shown in figure 42, next page). Watching the video clip made me wonder whether lymphocytes actually have the ability to lyse, destroy, or satisfactorily phagocytize spirochetes.

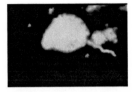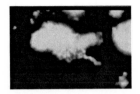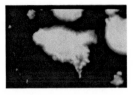

Figure 42 a, b and c (above, from left to right): A Lyme disease spirochete being engulfed by a lymphocyte.

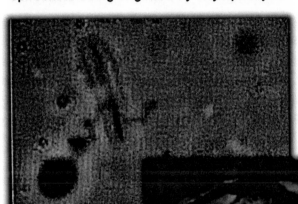

Figure 43:
An oral spirochete with granular bodies forming inside the cell membrane similar to what was shown in syphilis spirochetes.

Figure 44:
An active oral spirochete within the mucosal cell membrane.

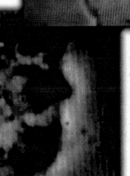

Figure 45: "Spore" appearing bodies, "inclusion bodies" or "phagosomes" within a lymphocyte taken from the blood during a root canal treatment. The blood came from the gingival sulcus that communicated between the tooth and a crown.

Whenever an immune cell ingests a pathogen, phagosomes or inclusion bodies are produced. Is it possible that the DNA of the spirochete remains intact inside the immune cell in the form of phagosomes? Or does the spirochete itself instead transform within the immune cell and produce a survival spore that remains stealthily housed within the cell cloaked as a phagosome? If the spirochete itself or enough of the DNA survives within the lymphocyte, in either scenario, can the altered form of the spirochete send signals within the now pathogenic host cell to other immune cells that the spirochete pathogen-destruction job was not completed by the original immune cell? If so, then in this manner, the immune system can become turned against itself and continue its attack upon the pathogen host-cell containing the spirochete DNA. Is such a phenomenon the definition of an autoimmune disease?

At the time when I theorized this point, I began looking for immune cells with phagosomes or inclusion bodies, especially lymphocytes. I observed the lymphocyte in figure 42, phagocytizing a Lyme disease spirochete; such a cell is likely to produce a phagosome. Maybe phagosomes are the key to understanding why spore-like bodies or spirochetal spores are found within the atherosclerotic plaque of blood vessels. The spirochete is ingested into the leukocyte and/or lymphocyte; however, before the immune cell can destroy the bacteria, the bacteria transforms into a spore. The resulting phagosome either goes unrecognized by the immune system or is attacked by the immune system because it is a host-cell for the spirochete. Once the immune system is finished with its localized assault, the membrane of the leukocyte pathogen host-cell eventually breaks down. This breakdown then contributes to the bulk of the fatty streak within the atherosclerotic plaque, thus depositing the spore into the atherosclerotic plaque lesion itself.

Two weeks prior to completing the final draft of this book, I was working on an endodontic (root canal treatment) procedure. It was bleeding from inside the access hole of the crown through which I needed to perform the root canal procedure. Later, I was able to identify the source of the bleeding. The bleeding was coming from periodontally diseased tissue, next to a pocket adjacent the tooth between the crown and the tooth. I was curious to see what type of bacteria was present in the blood.

A microscopic examination revealed a lymphocyte with several spores or phagosomes identical to the bodies I had found in other cases of periodontal disease and atherosclerotic plaque (figure 45, two pages prior). This was the first time, however, I had seen these bodies inside an immune cell in the gingival sulcus. It is beyond coincidence that the spores, phagosomes, or inclusive bodies contained within the lymphocyte were identical to those found in the atherosclerotic plaque and periodontal disease lesions. Do spirochetes use or hijack the immune cells in their lifecycle? The only remaining evidence needed to confirm this is DNA that positively identifies these spore-like bodies as spirochetal. However, until such evidence is available, we can only theorize that the spirochete is able to transform the immune cell so it becomes recognized as an invader by the immune system. Furthermore, I surmise that the spore form of the spirochete, rather than the active corkscrew form of the bacteria, is the injurious agent described by Fink and which hides inside of white blood cells. More research, however, is needed to get to the bottom of this issue.

The spore-like forms found within immune cells may also represent cell-wall-deficient forms of the spirochete, which are described by Lyme disease researchers. The spores I have identified in the mouth may represent such forms, but whether they are called cell-wall-deficient forms or spores may just be a point of semantics, because just as spores, cell-wall-deficient forms represent a protected form of the bacteria.

I have found that all of the morphological forms of spirochetes in the gingival sulcus are similar to those of the early syphilis spirochetes (figure 43, three pages prior), as well as Lyme disease spirochetes. What's more, live, active spirochetes have been identified as penetrating and living within the mucosal cells of the gingival sulcus (figure 44, three pages prior). Spirochetes, in general, all seem to have identical lifecycles and cause similar symptoms of disease.

Chapter 6
What Role Do Inflamed and Infected Teeth Play in the Labyrinth?

Inflammation is an important element in the progression of inflammatory arteriosclerosis and also helps to predict the future possibility of a heart attack. Thus, one clinical test performed by physicians that determines whether a patient has a predisposition for heart disease is a test for inflammation, which is called the CRP (C reactive protein).

In analyzing test results, it's important to know whether inflammation, when discovered, is a response to bacterial infection inside the endothelial lining of blood vessels or if it is the result of something else. The question must be asked: What role does non-specific inflammation play in the labyrinth? Non-specific inflammation caused by foci of infection that is distant from the atherosclerotic lesions is different from inflammation located at the site of an atherosclerotic lesion, but both can cause positive CRP test results. Inflammation caused by bacteria within the atherosclerotic lesion would indicate that the bacteria are in either an active or altered form, such as a cell-wall-deficient or spore that is able to send signals of its presence. However, inflammation present at a site distant from the location of the atherosclerotic plaque indicates that heart disease has been activated by signal chemicals produced by a distant bacterial infection.

Part of the theory I am proposing is that spirochetes present in the atherosclerotic plaque become active when they receive chemical signals as a result of inflammation present elsewhere in the body, even if the distal bacteria have nothing to do with the atherosclerotic lesion. Sources of inflammation in the mouth, for instance, can cause this to happen and are a result of conditions including periapical lesions associated with root canal–treated teeth, crestal bone loss caused by micro-leakage around dental implants, and periodontal disease, whether severe or mild. The CRP test for inflammation indicates one of two things: 1) that inflammation in general throughout the body predisposes patients to heart disease, or 2) only atherosclerotic lesions themselves produce the inflammation that predisposes a person to heart disease. In the first scenario, if generalized inflammation is important, then infections in the mouth may be the causative agents that signal distal bacteria in the atherosclerotic lesion to become active and cause a heart attack. If the second scenario is true and only the inflammation within the atherosclerotic lesion is important and is responsible for causing heart attacks and not inflammation in general, then inflammation in the mouth would cause false positives, if present, for heart disease. The oral source of inflammation and infection must be eliminated in either scenario.

Since there is a possibility that bacteria communicate with each other in the dental-atherosclerotic heart disease equation, let's review how they might accomplish this task. Dr. Bassler's work at Princeton University sheds much light on this issue. She discovered there needs to be a certain quorum, or concentration of bacteria, before they are able to perform certain activities. For instance, she found that bacteria produce small signaling molecules called auto-inducers, which synchronize group behaviors. The bacteria use quorum sensing to synchronize behavior such as pathogenicity (disease) and biofilm formation. Biofilms are essential and are implicated in the development of periodontal disease, and according to MacDonald, are present wherever spirochetes reside, i.e., in the brain lesions of Alzheimer's disease patients[56]. In her research, Bassler demonstrated how bacteria communicate with each other via these small RNA (genetic) chemical compounds, which are then sensed by a multitude of different interspecies bacteria[57] [58] [59] [60] [61] [62] [63]. She went on to postulate that these signals are important in the development of dental plaque, since these bacteria are highly organized and produce disease when they reach certain concentrations.

Even though the actual mechanism behind the quorum theory has not been understood, dentists have known about its consequences for many years. They know that if patients are put on a three-month recall schedule, periodontal disease bacteria do not have enough time to get organized and cause disease. Hence, my patients who are diagnosed with periodontal disease get placed on frequent recall schedules and are able to control their disease by coming in for recall visits.

It is logical that spirochetes also have the ability to communicate via quorum sensing. Inflammation caused by a small pocket of infection, foci of infection in the periodontium, the cratering of dental implants, or at the inflammatory infiltrate (infection) at the apex of an endodontically treated tooth, can signal spirochetes or bacteria distant to these locations to become active. In atherosclerotic plaque, when a spore becomes active, the body produces a localized inflammatory response within the plaque, with swelling and defensive infection-fighting cells present. This sets up the possibility for swelling within the plaque, as well as occlusion of the blood vessels and, subsequently, a heart attack. Furthermore, wherever inflammation exists, the tissue breaks down and provides nutrients for bacteria to consume.

The following cases will explore foci of infection within the oral cavity and which produce signals that activate distant bacteria, i.e., spirochetes. These small infections, in the present-day practice of dentistry, are not taken seriously and are not considered dangerous. The foci of infection theory was discredited in dentistry years ago because no evidence of clinical consequences as a result of such infections was found. The specialty of endodontics was approved by the American Dental Association more than thirty years ago, after years of bitter arguments over the foci of infection theory from many dental researchers and clinicians at the time. In many root canal–treated teeth, viable bacteria located in small pockets at the apex of the root are buried, ignored, and thought to be put to rest. Small numbers of dentists have protested the ignorance of these small infections ever since. The latest book written on the subject is *The Roots of Disease* by Robert Kulacz DDS and Thomas E. Levy MD, JD. These authors point out the problems with root canal–treated teeth. Dentistry will definitely have to revisit this issue because of the disease-creating potential of these small pockets of infection.

Since the recent arrival of implant dentistry, these small foci of infections are causing implant failures. If such infections can travel to an adjacent implant and cause failure, then these small bacterial infections, which are found in the periodontium or at the apex of a tooth, must be taken more seriously. The inflammation that they produce could be the trigger for acute atherosclerosis and a subsequent heart attack.

Nearby Foci of Infection that Caused Dental Implant Failures and Its Possible Role in Systemic Disease

The following patient histories are cases I have documented over the years, before I began using a microscope to study infected granulation tissue. Therefore, at this time, I have no exact evidence regarding which bacteria caused the problems in these cases. However, it is important to examine these cases because bacteria, whatever they are and wherever they are harbored in the body, cause problems. In the following cases, the bacteria caused either infection or failure of an adjacent dental implant. Most obvious and alarming to me over the years as I practice implant dentistry, are the bacteria associated with lesions at the apex, or next to the roots of teeth that have had previous endodontic (root canal) treatment. That infections occur here is evidence that the dental profession needs to change the way it understands and treats teeth that need endodontic therapy. Not all

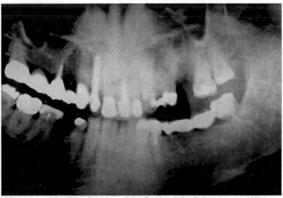

Figure 46: Patient with failed bridge needing dental implants.

endodontically treated teeth are bad; however, when a lesion is present at the apex of the tooth, treatment to eliminate the lesion and decontaminate the area must be performed, or else the tooth must be extracted and a dental implant placed.

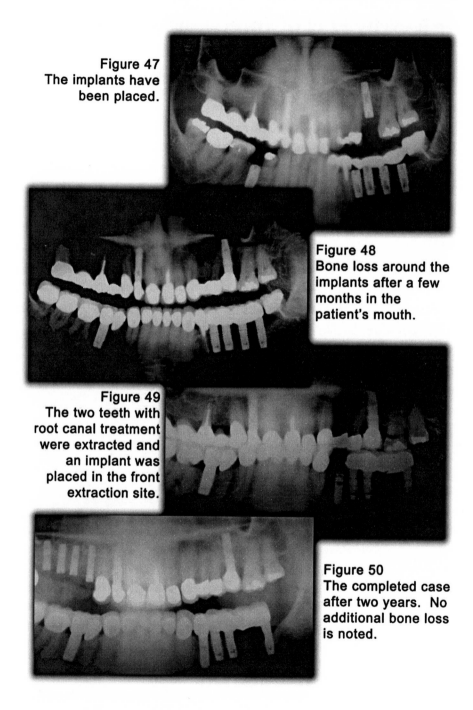

Figure 47
The implants have been placed.

Figure 48
Bone loss around the implants after a few months in the patient's mouth.

Figure 49
The two teeth with root canal treatment were extracted and an implant was placed in the front extraction site.

Figure 50
The completed case after two years. No additional bone loss is noted.

A prime example of the ability of small areas of infection to cause problems can be seen in a case that involved an infection associated with implants adjacent to two root canal–treated teeth. A fifty-three-year-old man came into my office with multiple missing teeth. One of the areas needing implants had a failed five-tooth bridge (figure 46, previous pages). From studying his mouth, it was evident that this upper-income, semi-retired patient had received state-of-the-art dental care and had excellent oral hygiene. I removed his failed bridge and placed four dental implants in the toothless area. There were two adjacent root canal–treated teeth, one in front of, and the other distal to, the newly placed implants. Neither of these teeth showed any X-ray evidence of infection. I also placed three additional implants in three separate quadrants of his mouth. Two of these quadrants did not have endodontically treated teeth present; however, the third had a root canal–treated tooth, but it was separated from the implant by two other natural teeth.

I placed the implants (figure 47), and at the end of five months, I finished them with crown and bridge restorations. The patient was then appointed for a six-month recall so I could check for any problems and perform a routine teeth cleaning. At the recall appointment, I noticed that the four implants that supported the fixed bridge exhibited bone loss ranging from one to seven millimeters (figure 48), as a result of infection. I suspected that the two adjacent root canal–treated teeth were the source of the infection.

With the patient's permission, I extracted these two root canal–treated teeth (figure 49). One of the two middle implants had experienced approximately 80 percent bone loss, so it was removed. As the surgery continued, the infected tissue from around the remaining implants was excised. Where the front root canal tooth was extracted, I placed a dental implant (figure 49) and, subsequently, a crown. Over the past two years, the patient has come into my office for follow-up visits (figure 50), and no further bone loss has been observed.

From this case, I learned:

1. No bone loss occurred around the other three single implants that were placed in the other three quadrants of the patient's mouth. These implants were not associated with any root canal–treated teeth adjacent to them. If periodontal disease had been present in this patient, then these implants would have been involved and there would have been bone loss. In this case, there was not. Even though I did not have microscopic evidence of periodontal disease, the above facts most likely ruled it out as a source of infection.

2. Bone loss occurred on implants that were immediately adjacent the root canal–treated teeth.

3. Once the root canal–treated teeth were removed, no further bone loss occurred around the remaining implants for at least three years (at the time that this book was completed).

4. Further research is needed to identify the causative bacteria associated with this infection and bone.

This case brings up that uncomfortable topic in dentistry that was once thought to be laid to rest many years ago; namely, the foci of infection theory, because it illustrates how small infections associated with root canal–treated teeth cause implants to fail. Also, documentation presented in this book as a result of previous articles provides ample evidence of problems with endodontically treated teeth adjacent to implants. What's more, if dental implants are affected, then other infectious problems in the body can potentially occur.

Many endodontically treated tooth problems that cause dental implant failure have been reported in the dental literature. Such failures are attributed to the following causes:

1. An infection in adjacent teeth at the bottom of a tooth root

2. Impingement by an implant that accidentally cuts into the adjacent tooth's root

3. Periodontal pathogens causing disease near an implant

4. Overheating the bone when drilling into it to place an implant

5. Implant contamination by periodontal bacteria and/or oral tissue cells, as a result of the gingiva being forced into the bone area where the implant is placed[64 65 66 67 68 69 70 71 72]. In this case, chronic infection, presumably resident in the vicinity of the adjacent endodontically treated teeth, allegedly invaded the bone around the implant, causing bone loss.

In the 1960 classic studies of Dr. Brynolf[73], cadavers were used to study root canal–treated teeth. These teeth were X-rayed and evaluated for evidence of radiolucent lesions at the apex or tip of the root deepest in the bone. The teeth were then cut from the bone with saws in block sections. The sections were treated and prepared for microscopic examination. Brynolf's evidence as a result of these examinations revealed that a lack of infection at the base of a root canal–treated tooth does not preclude inflammation or inflection at the apex of the tooth. She went onto say that 93 percent of root canal–treated teeth examined in cadavers had microscopic signs of inflammation (infection), presumably caused by bacteria in the area. Dr. Green et al[74] studied more cadavers in 1997 and characterized Brynolf's studies as questionable because of differences both in treatment techniques and methods of radiographic and histologic analysis that were being used at the time. Green reported that out of the 29 teeth examined, 15 had an alarming 52 percent histological evidence of inflammation, presumably infection associated with bacteria.

Reports of dental implant failures, along with the large percentage of periapical lesions associated with root canal teeth in cadavers, presents problematic evidence for the field of implant dentistry. How do we absolutely know which root canal teeth are bad before implants are placed? The risks to dentistry as a result of this ignorance as a whole are unimaginable, due to the liability that may now be attributed to dental clinicians because of recent findings relating dental infection to heart and other systemic diseases.

What Can Dentists Do about this and How Can the Public Protect Themselves When They Need Root Canal Treatment?

In today's cosmopolitan urban population, more than 51 percent of those with root canal–treated teeth probably have infections at the apex of their root. (This figure is higher than that reported by Green et al.) Although the percentage would probably not approach 93 percent, as reported earlier by Brynolf, Green's 52 percent (reported as a result of using what she refers to as modern methods) should be more than sufficient to alarm the dental profession. This figure represents millions of possible sources of dental implant infections. Even though the specific bacteria implicated in these implant failure case examples are unknown, whatever they are, they cause inflammation and bone loss. Any source of bacteria and chronic inflammation in the mouth may potentially relate to periodontal disease, as well as heart disease and other systemic diseases.

Over the years, I have noticed that at times, the bacteria associated with these infections are so virulent, that implants can be catastrophically lost within days of placement. Given they are virulent enough to cause bone loss and implant failure, it would also seem these bacteria have the capacity to cause more serious systemic problems. Blood tests for heart disease that detect inflammation in the body should alert dentists to search for a foci of infection in the mouth. Physicians need to alert dentists when they find increases in inflammation in the bloodstream, and historical evidence makes it obvious that there should be a major change in the way dentists treat abscessed teeth.

First, dentists treating abscessed teeth must take every possible step to sterilize the root canals of these teeth before completion. Dentists do not generally consider dentinal tubules as a source of infection to the body once the tooth is dead. The dentinal tubule[75] no longer has live nerves inside of it and becomes hollow, the size of a bacterium, after a root canal treatment. These vacant tubules, however, house bacteria and need to be sterilized during the endodontic procedure. Because of potential legal liabilities, even if the procedure is done correctly, verification that it has been done should also be documented because, while proof of sterilization was once considered the standard of care, it is no longer. The problem is that it is difficult, if not impossible, to sterilize the root canal and dentinal tubules of a dead tooth. Once the tubules or the tooth become contaminated with bacteria with resulting infection and bone loss, the root canal treatment procedure almost never completely eradicates the infection. This problem is a real dilemma for dentistry because, if this book is validated by dentists in general and the American Dental Association, then all existing root canal–treated teeth must be recalled and reevaluated for the smallest sign of periapical infection. If the infection cannot be eliminated by periapical surgery and decontamination, the tooth should be extracted. Before the arrival of dental implants, extraction of a tooth was a major problem for patients and was avoided by dentists. Today, when considering the negative long-term effects of inflammation on the body and its disease-producing potential, it is preferable that dentists extract questionable teeth and replace them with dental implants.

Another Source of Chronic Inflammation in the Mouth, Its Effect on Dental Implants, and How It Creates the Potential for Systemic Problems

Another problem in dentistry is a tooth with a crown that has no evidence of a problem, but which could, nonetheless, be necrotic and cause problems down the road. For example, in one of my patients, the elusive, asymptomatic, dead palatal root canal of an upper tooth with no prior evidence of infection (as ascertained by an X-ray) caused an adjacent implant failure. Many such peri-implant lesions have been reported. In the following case report, the loss of an implant resulted from an adjacent dead palatal root canal, which was difficult to diagnose.

The fifty-three-year-old female patient came to my office to have a tooth removed and an implant placed to replace the tooth (figure 51). Once an implant is placed, it must remain in the bone for approximately five months before it completely attaches itself to the bone. The process is called osseo-integration. When it is time to finish the implant, a second surgery is performed to uncover the implant and place an abutment that attaches to the crown. During my second surgery on this patient, I noticed she had an infection with a draining fistula next to the implant (figure 52). I completed a re-entry surgery to extirpate any infected granulation tissue. A 2- to 3-millimeter lesion at the tip of the implant was grafted using synthetic bone and an antibiotic. The remainder of the implant was solidly surrounded and integrated with what appeared to be dense normal bone. No acute bone infection was observed. Also, I found no visible track, which is when an infection drains to the surface of the gum through a fibrous hollow track pointing to a suspicious origin.

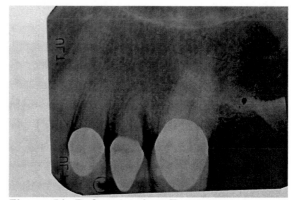

Figure 51: Before Implant Treatment; showing bone loss around middle tooth.

Having no other credible evidence, I then assumed the bacteria causing the lesion must have been forced into the peri-implant area during the implant installation procedure. The area healed normally, and I thought the problem had been resolved.

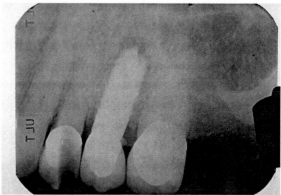

Figure 52: A peri-implant lesion on the implant caused by infection.

Soon after this patient's re-entry surgery, however, her infection began to drain once again. I then treated it locally with irrigation and put a slow time-released antibiotic

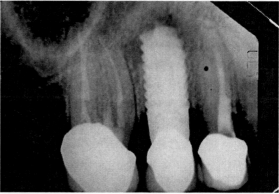

Figure 53: Implant area after two endodontic procedures were done on adjacent teeth.

into the infected area. After a short period of time, the infection did not resolve using this method, and I surgically examined the area to see if I had missed something. Nothing had changed, except that the augmentation material was absent, presumably due to chronic infection. I found no obvious reason for the drainage. Several weeks later, the patient again developed a small, draining fistula. Having ruled out problems with the implant itself, I then investigated the two adjacent teeth. Even though I had found no clinical or X-ray evidence of any problem with these teeth, with the patient's permission, I tested the vitality of the teeth, as doing so would help me to determine what the problem was. I used a high-speed carbide bur to cut a small round hole through the top of both crowns, and the bur penetrated into the dentin (sensitive inner part of the tooth) without an anesthetic. The front tooth (#5) tested non-vital; however, the patient experienced pain in her molar tooth (#3) when the drill penetrated the dentin. I diagnosed it to be alive and healthy. I placed a composite restoration in the #3 tooth and commenced endodontic treatment on tooth #5.

After I completed the endodontic treatment on tooth #5, the problem should have been solved. Unfortunately, shortly after this procedure, the patient once again developed a draining infection in the apical area of the implant. At that point, even though tooth #3 had tested alive and healthy, I immediately began to suspect there could be a problem with it, and that it might be what was causing the problem. Unlike tooth #5 and, in hindsight, this tooth had a slightly altered-suspect appearance on one of its roots when X-rayed. However, without any other evidence, and especially since the tooth had tested vital, I did not immediately suspect it.

When tooth #3 was opened, amazingly, a necrotic putrefying palatal pulp was found. The two buccal (toward the cheek) canals were completely filled with calcified material. I extirpated the dead tissue from the palatal canal intact with a barbed broach (a thin needle-shaped instrument that has many barbed projections from its surface to engage and remove nerve tissue from within the root canal). The dead tissue had a dark gray color and very fetid odor. The endodontic treatment was now completed (figure 53, two pages prior).

Since the diagnosis in this situation was so elusive and the final treatment resolution took several months, it was opted to remove the implant in this patient, so we would be assured of no future problems. All of the patient's symptoms resolved after the implant removal.

In this case, the loss of an implant resulted from a dead infected nerve canal, which required a very lengthy and difficult course to be discovered. Even though care must be taken to diagnose potential problems before implants are placed, in this case, such a diagnosis was not possible.

Chronic infection with resulting inflammation of asymptomatic teeth, especially in teeth that have been crowned, is probably more common than most dentists think. Implant dentists, fortunately, are becoming more aware of this problem because of cases of failed implants in the vicinity of such teeth. It has been well documented that the surfaces of dental implants are vulnerable to bacterial contamination during the early healing phase of the bone integration process. Experience has taught that the implant itself serves as a "dip-stick" or indicator of sub-clinical infection that might otherwise be difficult to diagnose in the oral cavity. In the above case, however, the implant procedure itself did not produce infection, since the infection problem associated with the implant occurred within five months of its placement. Infection that causes calcification of a root canal, such as that which occurred in this patient's two buccal canals, takes several years.

An additional source of this patient's infection could have been bacteria associated with the extracted tooth, which had been replaced along with the implant. The original tooth was loose; however, it had received root canal treatment several years prior to the patient's current treatment, but showed no evidence of periapical pathology. The socket was thoroughly cleaned before the implant was placed, and active infection was noticed after the implant was placed, even though no infection had previously been deemed present. The re-entry surgery ensured that the majority of the implant had osseo-integrated, thereby providing additional evidence that the source of the infection was probably not associated with the extracted tooth itself. Had it been so, the implant would not have integrated with the bone in the first place.

Even though others might disagree, I feel this patient's chronic infection existed long before the implant was placed, but the patient tolerated the infection until the implant was placed. Once the tip of the implant became contaminated by the bacteria in the bone, however, a more acute phase of infection occurred, which then resulted in a draining fistula. However, since the patient had already built up immunity to these bacteria over the years, an acute fulminating bone infection did not occur.

Generalized Inflammation

According to the Blaylock Wellness Report, *Inflammation: The Real Cause of Most Diseases*[76]; the most insidious killers of modern times share a common trait that precedes their devastating path of destruction; namely, inflammation. This report links inflammation to cancer, diabetes, heart disease, stroke, Parkinson's, and Alzheimer's disease. Inflammation is even implicated in depression, anxiety disorders and progressively debilitating chronic diseases, including Lou Gehrig's, multiple sclerosis, lupus, arthritis, and autism. In this report, no microorganism is proposed as a possible origin of inflammation. Instead, the inflammation is blamed on dietary factors and chemical environmental contaminants.

It has been documented in many places that dietary and environmental factors do, in fact, contribute to inflammation, just as bacteria do; however, it is my opinion that it is more likely that bacteria vastly contribute more to the condition of inflammation. Chronic infection in the oral cavity caused by one or more of the hundreds of different types of bacteria known to exist there is likely to affect the entire body, whether the infection is associated with an endodontically treated tooth, an asymptomatic necrotic nerve canal, crestal bone loss due to micro-leakage around dental implants, or periodontal disease. It is possible that these sources of inflammation trigger spirochete spores or cystic forms to activate within the atherosclerotic plaques found in the circulatory system, thereby causing swelling and cardiac incidences.

It is important to mention here that chronic inflammation over many years (15 to 20) has been reported to cause cancer. The mini-accesses or foci of infections caused by spirochete forms in dormant stage and that are located in tissue may have something to do with the future development of cancer resulting from chronic long-term inflammation. The spirochete is the initial stealth instigator of this cancer.

Medical literature also supports the fact that as people age, inflammation becomes increasingly present in the body, and when the long-term inflammation is in the mouth, advanced periodontal disease and tooth loss results. The final consequences of many years of inflammatory reactions to foci of infections are heart attacks, strokes, diabetes, and cancer. The villain responsible for these infections, oral spirochetes, may be the single most important player in diseases that cost the health-care system worldwide billions of dollars per year. But forget the financial cost; what is important is that this single bacterium, the spirochete, causes immeasurable pain and suffering to its victims, and eventually leads to a long and painful death in the last decades of life, as a result of the various inflammatory illnesses it causes.

Chapter 7
Multiple Missing Tooth Syndrome and How It Affects the Practice of Implant Dentistry

For many years, I have talked about and lectured on a subject I have defined as Multiple Missing Tooth Syndrome—for lack of a better term. Most of the patients who have come into my office for implant dentistry treatment to replace many missing teeth have multiple health problems, with symptoms that are strikingly similar, but subtler and chronic, to those found in syphilis and Lyme disease. Other symptoms are not as intuitively obvious until they are analyzed. If spirochetes can cause syphilis and Lyme disease, then why shouldn't oral spirochetes, which have been patronized by the dental profession, also have the ability to cause disease to the entire body, in a similar fashion to Lyme disease and syphilis? Periodontal disease is common among patients with multiple missing teeth; hence, it can be assumed they also have oral spirochetes that have had years to disseminate into the bloodstream and into the body's tissues.

Since periodontal disease is related to heart disease, it follows that those patients with heart disease often have many missing teeth. And, in fact, medical literature supports this theory[77] [78] [79]

⁸⁰. Patients with many missing teeth comprise a percentage of the patients within an implant dentistry practice, especially in a marketing practice that attracts patients who do not have a regular dentist. These patients seem to neglect their teeth more than patients who get regular cleaning and checkups. I'm not sure, however, that their dentists or the patients understand the full ramifications and implications of their diseases. Judging from the merits of the lawsuits that these patients bring against their implant dentists, it seems that some patients do not comprehend the difficulties that dentists face to complete an implant dentistry case successfully. Also, because these patients do not remember much about their consultations, the details of their visits must be written down, to prove to them that someone informed them of their treatment. Believe me, it is a monumental problem for implant dentists to treat such a group of patients.

Patients with multiple missing teeth resulting from chronic periodontal disease also have many different systemic problems. Their list of diseases includes:

1. Atherosclerosis, including patients with a history of:

   a. Heart disease. Some patients with this condition have had heart attacks, bypass surgeries, and stents placed by cardiologists. They are on blood thinners, aspirin, and cholesterol-lowering medications.

   b. High blood pressure. Patients with this condition take different types of high blood pressure medication.

   c. Strokes. Patients who have suffered a stroke have high blood pressure and take the same medications as mentioned above.

2. Dementia. Patients with this condition are probably in the early stages of Alzheimer's disease. For various reasons, their

condition makes implant dentistry almost unbearable for clinicians who do not understand their problem and its relationship to implant dentistry. First, they cannot reason properly, and most do not even realize they are mentally impaired. Secondly, if treatment doesn't go according to plan or when problems arise (and sometimes for no apparent reason), these patients develop completely off-the-wall theories regarding their treatment, and then insist that you listen and give credence to their theories. This makes the practice of implant dentistry unique among dentistry disciplines because implant dentists really need to be psychologists in order to practice.

3. Diabetes. Periodontal disease and diabetes are also related diseases. Many diabetic patients take insulin and drugs that stimulate the pancreas to produce more insulin and must control their condition through diet. As long as their symptoms are under control, implant dentistry can proceed normally.

4. Recurrent periodontal disease. Many of these patients have deep-seeded bacteria that are impossible to eliminate and that cause implant problems, as well as problems with any remaining teeth that they might have.

5. Cancer. Pancreatic cancer is linked to periodontal disease. Stomach cancer is linked to H. pylori. Long-term inflammation caused by micro-infections leads to cancer. The mechanism of the latter has been unknown until recently.

Once the relationship between these diseases and Multiple Missing Teeth Syndrome is understood, the relationship between the different spirochetal diseases becomes much more obvious. Spirochetosis, regardless of the type involved, produces the possibility for long-term inflammation and chronic disease. Inflammation caused by these spirochetes may also be the root cause of most chronic diseases, including arthritis and autoimmune and skin disorders, among many others.

Chapter 8
The History of, and Dentists' Frustration with, Periodontal Disease and What We Now Know about How to Treat It

For years, dentists have not been able to cure periodontal disease. And if they aren't able to understand the basics of this disease, how can they then relate it to such devastating systemic diseases such as those that we are discussing? In dentistry, it has generally not been known that spirochetes produce spores or some type of seeding or survival mechanism. Even when the immune system, as described earlier, engulfs spirochetes and packages them up inside its immune cells in the form of inclusive bodies or phagosomes, the spirochetal DNA may not be totally denatured. Indeed, it may still be active and able to signal a further inflammatory response. This reaction then produces chronic inflammation in the tissue, producing effects that have been mentioned in the preceding chapters.

The contents of this book may explain why, for so many years, dentists have been so excited about what they have discovered regarding the cause of periodontal disease, but subsequently disappointed when the disease returns after their best efforts. It explains why all the bacteria, including spirochetes, seem to show up in studies where participants are asked not to brush their teeth for prolonged periods of time. Progression of periodontal disease occurs in such patients, and eventually all the periodontal bacteria that cause severe gum disease can be isolated in their gum pockets, even when no apparent evidence of periodontal disease was present from the onset of the experiment. Spores or granules (some type of DNA packet), it would seem, are the only logical answer to the riddle of why oral spirochetes in periodontal disease show up when previously, no evidence of their presence was obvious. The three clinical cases reported in chapter five provide evidence for the existence of granular and cystic forms of spirochetes.

Yet, more study is needed to conclusively verify these findings, and Socransky points out this fact in his paper I referred to earlier. He also points out that initial enthusiasm for the hunt for etiological agents of periodontal disease slowly subsided during the late 1920s, so that by the mid-1930s, virtually no workers were involved in the quest anymore. He mentions that the researchers Belding and Belding eloquently lamented this issue in an aptly titled paper *Bacteria-Dental Orphans*. He also reports that from mid-1920 to the early 1960s, dentists' attitude toward the etiology of periodontal disease changed. They became more focused on facts such as trauma to the bite and disuse atrophy as a result of the modern diet. They thought that because of our soft diets, teeth were perceived as no longer being needed by the body; therefore, they developed periodontal disease. Bacteria were deemed as secondary in importance.

During the late 1950s, Socransky reports that a group of dentists, sarcastically referred to as the "plaque evangelists," placed heavy emphasize on plaque control. Plaque caused inflammation and inflammation was the cause of gum disease.

And so the cycle of discovery, forgetting, and rediscovery continues. The inflammation theory quoted earlier from Dr. Eugene S. Talbot MS DDS in 1899 was very accurate, but has been forgotten. In the face of reoccurrence of disease and disappointment because nobody has figured out the mystery of periodontal disease, clinicians have finally given up because it becomes an unwinnable battle. It's like being trapped in a labyrinth with no way out.

Chapter 9
The Course of Oral Spirochetal Illness

The oral spirochete that evokes an inflammatory response in the body seems to provide the crucial link between periodontal and atherosclerotic heart disease, as well as, between periodontal disease and diabetes, plaque-forming neurological diseases, and cancer. If oral spirochetes are a major player in the bacterial mix that causes the first gingivitis lesion (initial gum disease), then it is logical to believe these spirochetes are also the trigger for the complicated cascade of events that eventually result in serious illness. Bacteremias resulting from spirochetes enter the circulatory system and become seeded and rooted in various tissues of the body. Once entrenched there, they cause numerous inflammatory diseases as they transform and set themselves up for their next lifecycle journey into yet another host via a food-borne vector.

I postulate that the course of the oral spirochete disease can be described in the following manner:

1. Spirochete spores (cysts, spores, spherical bodies and/or granules) are deposited into the oral cavity through contact with some outside source, either a person or contaminated food.

2. They find their way into the gingival sulcus and remain there until conditions are favorable for their transformation into viable spirochetes that can cause periodontal disease. They may exist in the gingival sulcus as a spore or as a spiral non-disease producing active form for years, without causing inflammation. This period of latency provides a good opportunity for the dentist to diagnose (via microscope) and eliminate these early residents before they cause disease in the gingival sulcus and thereafter enter the circulatory system. Because once they are in the body, they become impossible to treat with modern medicine.

3. Periodontal infection then occurs, which can range in virulence from mild gingivitis to full-fledged Vincent's disease.

4. If the localized infection in the gums is not treated immediately with chemicals or antibiotics, the viable spirochetes then enter the bloodstream during a bacteremia (caused by chewing, dental cleaning, periodontal probing that causes bleeding or any other gum tissue manipulation) and disseminate throughout the body. In the case of atherosclerosis, the spirochetes can easily enter the endothelial lining of the blood vessel at multiple locations, resulting in multiple, multi-sized lesions that can be observed by modern diagnostic ultrasound units. These lesions are probably located throughout the body's circulatory system and are caused by a multitude of spirochetes penetrating and residing in the endothelial lining over a lifetime of episodic periodontal disease.

5. The body's defense mechanisms attack the active spirochete form within the endothelial lining. However, during the attack, the spirochete transforms to different forms, whether inside an immune cell or within the plaque itself, to produce what looks like phagosomes or inclusive bodies. The spirochete either produces spores, or converts into cyst or cell-wall-deficient-forms, which are eventually left behind in the atherosclerotic plaque deposits. The spores or other forms remain there until a favorable condition (anything that results in a depression of the immune system or inflammation) exists to transform the spores into viable spirochetes once again.

6. In the case of Vincent's disease, and in the worst-case scenario, the spore or other dormant form transforms into an active form and the body attacks the bacteria yet again, causing inflammation, swelling of the atherosclerotic lesion, and possibly perforation of the endothelial lining of the blood vessel. This results in blood clots and arterial blockage and sets the stage for a heart attack.

7. In situations where oral spirochetes find themselves in other tissues of the body, any chronic inflammatory disease, such as Alzheimer's disease, and other plaque-forming neurological disease, autoimmune diseases, skin disorders, and ultimately, cancer, can be caused by the spirochete foci of chronic infection initiator.

Knowledge of this new discovery should stimulate research into a possible cure for these insidious oral spirochetal diseases. If the theory I propose proves to be true, then a massive effort by the medical and dental community should be mounted so we can find a way to interrupt and curb this elusive, multiform enemy. Understanding these bacteria's ability to transform into a protected spore, cell wall deficient, or cyst form without being destroyed when treated with conventional antibiotics is of paramount importance to both physicians and dentists. Even when attacked and engulfed by the immune cells, they seem to have the ability to consolidate their DNA into a protective form within the attacking cell. I theorized that if spirochetes were the culprits in heart disease, then their spores would be present in the atherosclerotic plaque of blood vessels. And indeed, the final piece of the puzzle was put into place when, through the use of my microscope, I found identical, morphologic spore-like forms in atherosclerotic plaque taken from the aorta. These spores have a unique morphological signature and their identity is all but unmistakable. DNA analysis is the final proof, but that requires large research grants, to which I do not have access, as of yet.

In my extensive research, discussed earlier, I also found that the veterinarian literature reported that similar, if not identical, spirochetes have been found in cattle and sheep. Therefore, it is likely that the transmission of spirochetes to humans via food-borne vectors is also possible.

From the convincing data presented here, it is evident that we have a huge problem because spirochetes are able to conceal themselves by existing in a latent or resting state until conditions in the body become favorable for their reemergence. This is part of their survival strategy and the reason why they can cause severe damage. There are no known methods to kill their spore-like bodies, and they seem to be protected from antibiotics. Thus, they must be able to sense when conditions are favorable for reemergence. Some of these conditions include when a person has periodontal disease or depressed immune function, small or large levels of inflammation in the mouth or body, a change in pH, and/or a surgical or traumatic wound. In an opportunistic way, the bacteria seem to be able to seek out their inflammatory target and infect it. Hence, the treatment and cure for this disease appears to be an almost insurmountable task.

Chapter 10
Today's Prevention and Treatment of Periodontal Disease: Is It Enough?

What is being done to find a cure for periodontal disease and eliminate the bacteria that cause it? The answer is not enough, unless there are treatable symptoms of disease. Then the symptoms are treated, but not the root cause. In the case of periodontal disease, even then, and except for the practitioners with microscopes, those who treat periodontal disease rarely ever attempt to eliminate the bacteria that cause it before signs and symptoms appear. Even the "microscope dentists" probably do not examine every patient who comes to their office when evidence of disease is not apparent. Most dentists only treat active disease and do not even look for spirochetes in those patients who don't have symptoms. And if they do, do they know about spherical bodies, cysts, cell-wall deficient, and other spirochetal forms? Dentists only treat the patients who show clinical signs and symptoms of periodontal disease, once the disease becomes active. By the time dentists treat diagnosable periodontal disease, it is usually too late because, once disease has occurred and the first gingivitis is present, spirochetes have already gained entrance to the body to cause systemic disease. And the longer periodontal disease is allowed to remain in the gums, the more spirochetes gain access to the body and become embedded into the endothelial lining of blood vessels. Then there is more chance for heart disease and other systemic diseases.

In dentistry, prevention is the key since, in my opinion, these bacteria gain access to the body through the gateway of the diseased gingival tissue. Since contamination of the gingival sulcus can occur at any time, via oral transmission or food contamination, the active spirochetal bacteria and its spores must be removed from the gingival sulcus before they reach whatever number and/or other combination of other bacteria that is necessary to cause disease. Any small source of inflammation must be eliminated, including residual periapical lesions at the tip of root canal–treated teeth, inflammation associated with crestal bone loss from around dental implants because of micro-leakage, and basically any form of periodontal disease, no manner how slight. Periodontally diseased granulation tissue must also be eliminated aggressively, whether surgically, by laser, or non-surgically. Most commonly, a combination approach should be used.

Once a patient is infected, however, there seems to be a window of opportunity; that is, a time period in which spirochetes can be effectively eliminated from the gingival sulcus before they cause periodontal disease and gain entrance into the circulatory system. This refractive time period should be taken advantage of by developing methods of diagnosis and treatment to use during this time, so the bacteria may be eliminated before they cause systemic disease. There are oral hygiene methods discussed later in this chapter and chapter 11 that dentists and patients can begin using today to help initiate the prevention of heart disease, which causes more deaths in the industrialized world than all other diseases combined.

The first stage of an oral spirochete infection causes initial gingivitis, a condition that is characterized by slightly swollen red periodontal tissue. These inflamed tissues bleed easily when brushed. Traditionally, this has been treated with good oral hygiene. However, considering the fact that such an infection can cause the development of heart disease, more aggressive treatments might be warranted; but any manipulation of the tissue during diagnosis and treatment that could cause a bacteremia should be avoided. Irrigation of the tissue with a bactericidal agent should be employed prior to any dental treatment to avoid causing such bacteremias.

Unfortunately, there is no known cure once the spirochetes have disseminated throughout the body and reached the tertiary spore or cyst stage. The only way to fight the disease when it reaches this stage is to keep the immune system strong by practicing good oral hygiene, physical health and nutrition, not smoking, maintaining good mental health and attitudes, and by appropriately handling stress. This will keep the spores from transforming in the face of what they would perceive as an opportunity to once again multiply and cause problems.

Preventing contamination of the gingival sulcus is another matter altogether and everyone should be involved in this process. A quick and easy microscope-screening exam should be performed and whenever spirochetes or their spores are identified, a simple bactericidal irrigation of patient's gingival sulcus should be performed. This is especially important for children. There are any numbers of bactericidal chemicals that can be used for this process, including diluted bleach, Chlorohexidine, and baking soda solution. All of these will kill any active pathogenic organisms.

Just out of curiosity, I researched medical literature to discover whether there was any evidence that toothpaste might help to fight periodontal disease. Without exception, in each and every scientific paper that I analyzed, toothpastes with sodium or stannous fluorides, Triclosan, or any combinations of these chemicals, only reduced the presence of bacteria, but never came close to eliminating them[81]. Therefore toothpaste, even though it tastes good, is not effective for eliminating the disease, only maintaining it.

Mouth washes, even though they are good for killing bacteria immediately after kissing someone, do not penetrate down into the gingival sulcus and therefore, do not eliminate the bacteria. Studies have shown that while mouthwashes can reduce gum disease, they cannot eliminate it.

Brushing and flossing are ineffective at eliminating these bacteria for one obvious reason; they simply cannot get to the bottom of the gingival sulci where the bacteria reside. Like mopping the floor with a wet mop without detergent, brushing your teeth only moves the bacteria around but does not eliminate them.

The only real hope of controlling periodontal disease is by eliminating the bacteria that cause it. This book proposed that the major player in this disease is the spirochete, and is based on the premise that spirochetal infections are extremely difficult, if not impossible, to eliminate once they gain a foothold in the body, and for this reason, infection prevention is the real key to health. So how do you get rid of spirochetes from the gingival sulcus? I have demonstrated in this book that antibiotics are not the solution; they only postpone the problem. Initially, when spores get into the gingival sulcus, they must be flushed out with an irrigation device with a cannula, in order to get to the bottom of the sulcus.

Chapter 11
Treating Periodontal Disease in Its Early Stages

The gingival sulcus should be irrigated with an antimicrobial chemical prior to any dental treatment, especially prior to periodontal probing, which measures the depths of periodontal pockets around the teeth and prophylaxis. There is recent evidence from the *New England Journal of Medicine* that aggressive periodontal disease treatment causes the endothelial lining of arteries in patients with atherosclerotic heart disease to perform worse, before it gets better[82]. This is presumably because of the fact that aggressive periodontal treatment causes bacteremias; therefore, the endothelial lining initially reacts to these bacteria in the blood by decreasing blood flow, before long-term benefits of periodontal treatment, resulting in better endothelial performance, are realized. Once the bacteria have been cleared and the periodontal disease is under control, only then does the endothelial lining perform better.

My treatment regimen comprises a series of three appointments following the initial diagnosis and treatment planning session. During these appointments a laser is first used to eliminate the lining of the gingival sulcus, and then irrigation devices with thin cannulas are used to deliver antimicrobial chemicals to the bottom of the gingival sulcus. These devices, along with the chemicals, effectively reach and kill active bacteria as they flush out spores.

Treatment Appointment #1: (We call this first appointment Life Guard #1.) This first irrigation is performed during the second week a patient is on antibiotics. Patients who have been diagnosed with severe periodontal disease, either with a microscope or in combination with a bacterial culture, which is sent to the Oral Microbiology Testing Service at the University of Southern California, are placed on a combination of laboratory-recommended antibiotics or standard antibiotics that have been proven effective for killing the oral bacteria. The reason why I still use antibiotics during this first appointment is to prevent any bacteremias during the aggressive debridement (cleaning out) of calculus and plaque from under the gums. After this deep cleaning, I use a CO_2 laser—in my office I use a Deka Ultra-speed soft-tissue laser. There are other lasers used that are also effective, i.e., Diode lasers and the Millennium Laser. I perform a gingival curettage, which involves removing the lining of the gingival sulcus, to eliminate any spores that might be in the gingival tissue itself. So far this has been very effective; however, since this treatment is new, more time is needed to fully assess this method. I then irrigate the gingival sulcus with Peridex (0.12 % Chlorhexidine).

Treatment Appointment #2: (Life Guard #2) The patient returns one week after the initial visit, and once again, I perform a bacterial examination using the microscope. At this point, in the vast majority of my cases, mobile bacteria can no longer be seen in the microscopic field. I then perform an ultrasonic cleaning and second irrigation, using diluted sodium fluoride (the same used for topical decay prevention). It has been well documented[83], that fluoride is effective against certain bacteria[84] [85] [86] and induces re-mineralization of incipient decay. It is also thought to fill in dentinal tubules. The problem of bacterial re-population of the sulci may be due in part to exposed dentinal tubules[87] (these are the millions of microscopic channels in dentin) because tubules are a perfect place for bacteria to hide, given their size. The fluoride treatment is thought to help plug these tubules to prevent and kill resident bacteria. Antibiotics cannot penetrate and kill bacteria located in these tubules, while fluoride can.

Treatment Appointment #3: (Life Guard #3) I check the bacteria once again and perform a third irrigation. This irrigation uses diluted Stannous fluoride (another topical fluoride treatment used for decay prevention). My personal, but not published, research completed in the early 1970s demonstrated that sodium fluoride and stannous fluoride have a synergistically positive effect when used together. Therefore, a second, but different, stannous fluoride solution is used. The fluoride ion creates a hostile environment for bacteria in the gingival sulci, and its effects remain there for a long period of time. The compound Stannous-fluoro-phosphate $(Sn_3F_3PO_4)$[88] [89] [90] [91], a product formed during the stannous-fluoride reaction, is very insoluble and remains compounded in the tooth structure within the sulcus to inhibit bacterial growth.[92] So far, and in my experience, a combination of three irrigations with three different chemical regimens has eliminated the mobile bacteria in the sulci and has not allowed for any re-colonization.

In addition to the treatments patients receive in the dentist's office, they should also irrigate their mouths daily with a Water-Pik™, Hydro floss™, or Viajet Pro™ type device. This is essential for long-term care of the mouth and for preventing re-contamination of bacteria. Once the patients have irrigated the gingival sulcus using one of these devices, they should brush their teeth with a baking soda and salt mixture wet with peroxide. This is prepared using one half cup of baking soda mixed with one teaspoon of salt. Patients wet the toothbrush with the peroxide, dip it into the salt mixture, and then brush their teeth by working the mixture into the gingival sulcus. These strategies, when used together at night, have proven to be a long-term solution to prevent the re-population of the gingival sulcus with spirochetes that result from food or oral contamination. Thus, this regimen is successful for daily maintenance of a healthy mouth. I have also found that patients who are compliant in this hygiene method do not have plaque on their teeth when coming in for their three- or six-month checkups. There is no plaque to look at under the microscope, which is the ultimate goal patients should strive for.

Another successful treatment is found in the use of long-acting antibiotic powders, such as tetracycline (Arestin®), or antibiotic pastes that are placed deep into the gingival sulcus to eliminate the problematic bacteria. It is thought that this type of treatment has the potential to kill spirochetes before they transform into spores or other forms, and is used as a first step in periodontal treatment by many dentists.

Additional methods of treatment will be developed which may be even more effective than this one, i.e., electro-magnetic pulse devices. When patients have gum disease, the most effective way of removing causative bacteria may be through a combination of all methods available, including common periodontal surgery, the use of surgical lasers to remove all granulation tissue, along with the later non-surgical use of irrigations in the gingival sulcus, using several chemical agents.

In Summary

The purpose of this book was twofold; first, to propose a new theory that explains the relationship between periodontal and systemic disease, especially heart disease; and second, to stimulate research and funding to prove the postulates and theory of this work.

The following describes a summary of my conclusions, based on the main points of this book.

1. Almost everyone (about 80 percent of the population) seems to have the spirochetal bacteria that can lead to periodontal and heart disease. The theory presented explains, among other things, how many debilitating chronic diseases, with this one initiating cause, become stealth killers after many years of dormant coexistence in our body's tissue.

2. Periapical lesions at the apex of endodontically treated teeth need to be eliminated. It appears from the medical literature that more than 50 percent of root canal–treated teeth have these lesions. Dentists must evaluate these teeth as to whether they can be saved in a healthy manner, otherwise these teeth must be extracted and replaced with dental implants.

3. For patients contemplating having a root canal treatment completed on an abscessed tooth, they must be sure that the dentist can eliminate the infection before the root canal procedure is finished, otherwise have the tooth extracted and replaced with a dental implant.

4. Dentists need to eliminate the bacteria that were once considered to be indigenous and normal to the gingival sulci. My review of the medical literature clearly demonstrates that spirochetal bacteria are likely to be these bacteria and the culprit in chronic inflammatory diseases. Everyone should have their gingival sulci screened, and if spirochetes or spores are recognized, then treatment with various methods, including irrigation, should be performed on a regular

schedule until it is proven that these bacteria have been eliminated. Treatment should also be performed on a macro-level until the bacteria are eliminated in the population worldwide. Also, these pathogenic microbes should be eradicated in the gingival sulcus by irrigation prior to any dental procedure.

5. There doesn't seem to be any cure for spirochetal illnesses once the bacteria disseminates into the body. Only an excellent immune system with resulting mutual coexistence with the bacteria can protect us from these bacteria and give us a long healthy life, until a method for denaturing spores is found.

In a medical environment where we have the benefit of being able to prescribe antibiotics, we may have become lax in our efforts to eliminate bacteria associated with abscessed teeth. This laxity needs to stop. We have an incurable disease that can be prevented, but only with extreme diligence and hard work. Since spirochetes can be transmitted orally from person to person via spores and possibly also through contaminated food, dentists need to monitor spirochetal bacteria frequently, using a micro-scope. Since morphological, identical spores have been identified in the gingival sulcus and the atherosclerotic lesions in blood vessels, further research should be conducted at multiple institutions in order to verify this observation. Indeed, research funds need to be appropriated so that this excellent work may be continued, as soon as possible. Millions of lives are counting on it. By understanding the spirochetal bacteria life forms that are causing the problem, treatments can be developed to cure the disease.

Chapter 12
Epilogue

The Common Denominator: Oral Spirochetosis

This book has been in progress for almost two years. After the discoveries and coming to a new understanding of periodontal disease and its relationship to systemic disease, I have observed the consequences of this spirochete-systemic disease relationship in some key patient cases. I realize this is strictly anecdotal evidence; however, the observations made in these several cases can add valuable information in the continued study of this relationship between oral spirochetosis and systemic diseases.

Patients' names have been changed to protect their privacy. However, with permission, most of these patients would be more than happy to discuss their situation with inquirers.

Board Member of a Prestigious Local San Diego Hospital has a Heart Attack: Two years ago, an affluent 50-year-old Caucasian male came to my office for implant dentistry. He had multiple missing teeth with some severely decayed remaining teeth with periodontal disease. Steven was a successful businessman who had taken an already established industry and used his innovation skill and efficiency to streamline production. He built new stores in several cities with his new model to the extent that he made millions of dollars for his efforts. Because of his innovative skill, he was invited to become involved with building a new hospital in China. The hospital proved successful, and others are in the planning stage there. He serves on the board of directors of a prestigious San Diego hospital.

I have had the opportunity to treat many top executives from many large successful companies in the San Diego area. These top executives are hard-driving; they work long hours and are charismatic. However, I have noticed that in this high-stress environment their teeth have been neglected and taken a beating. They especially have severe periodontal disease.

This was the scenario for Steven. Even though he was successful, his teeth were all but lost to periodontal disease. He did not even look healthy. I did a microscopic examination on him and found the usual severe bacteria-appearing pattern that is common with these executives. I saw many fast-moving spirochetes. During his treatment, we became friends so I was able to talk with him extensively about his condition and the writing of this book. He learned more than the average patient about his condition as I treated him during the months in my office. This information I gave him would later prove to save his life.

I immediately placed him on the Life Guard program and the hygiene methods I have described in Chapter 11. When I was satisfied with his progress and home care, I placed many implants to restore his teeth. He received fixed ceramic crown and bridge, which simulates natural teeth. He was delighted with the results.

About halfway into his treatment, he arrived at my office with an incredible story. The main headquarters for his business is in a Midwestern city. Therefore he commutes on weekends to San Diego. He loves his beachfront home and enjoys the wonderful weather and living environment. In dramatic terms, he told me that while traveling back to San Diego; he had severe heart pain, sweats and the feeling of an elephant foot on his chest. These were unmistakable signs of a heart attack.

Steven further told me that he absolutely knew what was happening to him, but he didn't want to tell the flight attendant for fear they would land the airplane at the nearest city with a hospital. He wanted to return to San Diego where he could be treated at the hospital where he served on the board. He said that when I had told him that he most likely had heart disease, he studied heart disease and knew exactly what to do if he had a heart attack and how to survive it. I did tell him that based on the fact that he had severe periodontal disease, he was a candidate for a heart attack.

As a result of this knowledge, he coughed his way back to San Diego sweating profusely every minute of the way. Coughing is a method that helps pump blood through a heart when the heart is compromised during an attack. He told me that the remaining two hours of the flight were the longest of his life. Once the plane landed he informed the flight attendants of his life-threatening condition. He was rushed to his requested hospital.

A world-renowned cardiologist placed a stent in the problematic artery of his heart and he suffered no ill effect from postponing his treatment. However, the doctor said that thirty more minutes and he would have not survived his heart attack.

Now that Steven is finished with his treatment, I can definitely say that he looks much healthier. He tells me that he feels great now that his periodontal disease is under control. He has committed to daily oral hygiene and a healthier lifestyle.

Steven told me that he attributes his survival to me. If I hadn't told him of his possible heart disease, he wouldn't have studied the subject and wouldn't have known what to do. Patients, who are successful and work too much and have bleeding gums, loose teeth, or many missing teeth because of gum disease, should immediately seek the care of a dentist. They need to get their periodontal disease under control to prevent such an incidence that Steven endured. He was lucky. He lived. Many would not survive such a heart attack.

Lyme-Like Antibiotic Treatment Saved This Patient's Life: When concepts that were not understood in the past, but become evident after a paradigm shift in thinking occurs, problem patients from the past who are examples of these concepts leap to the forefront of your consciousness. Such a patient is Mr. Michael Jones. Michael is a striking example of how similar Lyme disease is to periodontal disease. When I treated Michael years ago, I had no idea the extent and severity of Lyme disease; additionally, it was long before I made the correlations between the two diseases.

After writing this book, which involved becoming knowledgeable in the treatment of Lyme disease, Michael's case ran through my mind time and time again. Michael is a 70-year-old patient who had a long history of episodic infection around his dental implants. He also suffered from prostate cancer and sought alternative treatments to cure his condition. He did not want surgery to remove the organ. His condition almost killed him, and if it weren't for the "grace of God" and a talented infectious disease physician, he would be dead. He was about as close to the "gates of heaven" as any patient I have treated—and he survived.

Michael is committed to spreading the word of his condition and the treatment that saved his life.

Michael came to my office fifteen years ago for dental implants. He received upper and lower implants with a removable denture that snapped onto a bar that was secured to the implants. This was a life-changing procedure for Michael—since he previously couldn't enjoy a meal because of his ill-fitting dentures. Patients, including Michael, silently suffer their fate, become depressed, and definitely do not enjoy life. You never hear about these "toothless" patients because they are so embarrassed that they failed in their lives and lost their teeth. Even wives keep their dentures secret from their husbands. When treating these patients, we are many times asked not to talk about their treatment with their spouses.

In Michael's case, he had a beautiful, young wife; he was a young thinker and was not ready to become a dormant sedimentary senior citizen. He wanted to be active, to socialize, and to go out to a fine restaurant and enjoy good food. He had been successful in his life, so why not. The "why not" was that he couldn't enjoy eating with his denture. Not only did he lose all of his teeth, but he also had lost most of the bone in his upper jaw and his denture would loosen and fall down every time he bit into anything. To him, denture adhesives were disgusting. He was silently miserable and was determined to find an answer to this disruption in his otherwise exciting life.

Michael researched dental implants, which in the late eighties, were a new procedure and not many dentists were offering this service. He came to my office for a dental implant consultation and was given a treatment plan that included both upper and lower implants to stabilize a removable over-denture. These appliances are the most life-changing appliances I have ever made. Changing these patients' lives is without question the motivating force of my life.

Shortly after we completed his implant treatment, Michael reported to me that he had been diagnosed with prostate cancer. He was determined to cure this cancer without surgery and began his long quest to conquer this new adversary and deterrent to his newly achieved wonderful "toothed" life. This life included, for the first time in many years, menus of great food.

During the next ten-year time frame, Michael came to see me at least three occasions with infections around his dental implants. At the time, I treated patients who had infections, such as Michael's, by taking a culture of the infection and sending it to Dr. Slots at the Microbiology Testing Laboratory at the University of Southern California. The laboratory would culture the sample and do what is called a sensitivity test of the microorganisms to antibiotics. They would then send the antibiotic recommendations back to me with the report detailing the type of bacteria present. In all three reports I did, no spirochetes were reported present in any of the cultures. My understanding of the reports back them was if there is no report of spirochetes, there were no spirochetes. Today, I know differently. As I discussed in this book, the laboratory only tests for one of the sixty known species of spirochetes in the mouth. I wish I had known then what I know today. All the signs and symptoms of this patient as I understand the disease today were of oral spirochetosis.

Each time he came in with an infection, I sent off the culture to the microbiology laboratory and treated Michael with the recommended antibiotics and he would respond favorably and recover from the infection. During this timeframe, Michael was reading and studying ways to cure his prostate cancer. He came into my office regularly for hygiene checkups and cleanings, and each time he arrived, he reported the latest treatment for the prostate cancer.

On one occasion, he came into my office to say he was on laetrile, a controversial drug made from the pits of apricots that is purported to cure cancer. Supposedly, the active ingredient in laetrile is cyanide. Since Michael was intelligent and observant, he wanted me to see that since he had been on the laetrile, he had completely cured the infection around his implants. Being skeptical, I didn't take much regard of his observation until I did an examination. To my surprise, Michael had made the correct observation. The tissue around the implant was perfect. I've thought about that observation several times since that day: Is cancer caused by infection, i.e., his prostate cancer? Do small amounts of cyanide kill the microorganism that causes cancer? Why would laetrile cure cancer? Why is it effective against dental infection? All of this questions are apropos to the theories of this book.

The last episode in Michael's infection came about four years ago. His upper implants were loose, and the lower implants had about one-third bone loss. After placing Michael on one more regiment of antibiotics, I removed the upper implants and did a revision surgery on the lower implant to save them. After several postoperative checkups and remaking his upper denture, I didn't hear from Michael for about a year.

Michael came in not looking well. He said that during that year he had had an infection in his heart and had major heart reconstruction. The physician only gave him a 5 percent chance of surviving the surgery. He said he was so grateful to God to have survived the ordeal. The surgery included building a new heart valve with a pig heart valve. The surgery was successful; however, the physician was concerned because tests showed he still had infection in his body that she feared would reinfect his heart and damage the new pig valve. The physician requested that Michael return to my office to check his lower implants to see if the infection was coming from that source. I checked the implants and determined that they were infection-free, and the tissue was healthy around these implants. Michael thanked me and I didn't hear from him for several months.

When I saw him again, he looked remarkably better. His color was back, and he was his usual cheery self. He then related to me that his astute infectious disease physician in an effort to mitigate the chronic infection in Michael's body had infused him forty times with IV Rocephin during a several month period of time. This treatment cost the insurance company $50,000. Rocephin is a group of drugs called cephalosporin, and it's used to treat severe or life-threatening bacterial infections. The physician persisted with the infusion until Michael's inflammation tests showed no signs of infection remaining in his body. At the time, Rocephin was a novel, expensive drug that was only used in these severe infection situations. Today, it's more common and not as expensive.

Back then, I had no idea about the treatment of chronic Lyme disease. I knew about Lyme disease and that it was a spirochete, but nothing about its chronic infection potential. Today, I do. One of the most successful treatments of chronic Lyme disease is long-term IV infusions of Rocephin. What a coincidence!

In my heart, I know the origin of Michael's infection. It came from the periodontal disease that caused the loss of Michael's teeth in the first place. This infection in turn caused the multiple infections of Michael's implants that I was unsuccessful in treating because of lack of knowledge in treating chronic spirochetosis. This infection then caused the loss of the upper implants. The same infection then caused the infection in Michael's heart that almost caused his death. Also, I might add, what do you think of the possibly that this infection also caused his prostate cancer? I would think there's a good chance.

Michael now comes in every three months to check his lower implants for the less amount of infection. My observation has been since his infusion with Rocephin, I cannot find any plaque around his lower implants. It has been almost two years since his treatment with the antibiotic and still no plaque. I know he is now motivated to do his hygiene every day, but few patients ever report for a follow-up examination who do not have at least a little plaque. He had none.

This knowledge of chronic spirochetosis leaves me with a frustration in the treatment for oral spirochetosis. In oral infections, we rarely treat with antibiotics for more than two weeks. For Michael, my antibiotic treatments in the past were not long enough to rid him of his chronic oral spirochetosis. If I take the lead in dentistry and start treating oral spirochetosis with long-term IV antibiotics, I can already hear the criticism I would receive from my colleagues. When you study chronic Lyme disease, it is still extremely controversial. Only recently has long-term antibiotics been accepted by the physicians. I think my next move in this search for a treatment for chronic periodontal disease will include consultations with infectious disease physicians. I just can't conceive, at least for the near term, my placing patients on IV long-term antibiotics. Armed with this knowledge, new treatment regiments need to be devised for this problem.

Alzheimer's Patient Case: About two years ago, Mary, a 60-year-old Caucasian patient, presented to my office with persistent heavy calculus accumulation around her teeth, especially on her lower front teeth. I performed a microscopic examination on her that revealed mobile bacteria—but no spirochetes. She reported that she had been to several dentists to try and get control of this heavy calculus accumulation, with no success. I recommended that she use an irrigator every night before bedtime and use baking soda and salt on a toothbrush wet with hydrogen peroxide. I then cleaned her teeth and scheduled her a follow-up to evaluate her condition in two weeks.

To my dismay, she again had heavy accumulations of calculus on her teeth. I worked with her on brushing techniques and cleaned her teeth. Again, I appointed her for another follow-up to evaluate her progress. She did do a better job, but all too much calculus had again accumulated on her teeth. I determined that I should clean her teeth once a month. As time went on, she always needed further cleaning. I knew that it was a hopeless case and she would need frequent follow-up cleanings to maintain her dental health. Several follow-up microscope examinations still revealed no spirochetes.

About one year into this treatment she mentioned that her husband, Albert, had Alzheimer's disease and had very bad breath. He was still ambulatory and still functional, but definitely had severe memory problems. Since he always accompanied her to her cleaning appointments, I requested of her to bring him into the operatory so I could check his bacteria. Albert's examination revealed extremely active mobile bacteria with what can best be described as a "furious-type" of movement on the microscopic slide at 1000X. He had very fast-spinning spirochetes of differing sizes, trichomonads (parasites that look like little mice running around the sample), and multiple different-appearing motile rods. He had plaque coating all of his teeth, which could best be characterized as extremely poor oral hygiene.

Mary reported to me that Albert had once been placed on an antibiotic in the past for an unrelated infection. She told me that when he was on these antibiotics, his Alzheimer's disease symptoms had drastically improved. However, when she requested that the physician allow him to remain on the antibiotics, he refused and said it was just coincidental that he improved during the antibiotic regiment. I agreed to treat Albert's periodontal disease and placed him on the Life Guard treatment, which included antibiotic treatment for two weeks.

When the patient returned for his second Life Guard treatment, one-and-a-half weeks into the antibiotic treatment, Mary reported this finding. They were out shopping for food at the grocery store when she realized she had forgotten her grocery list. Albert, without skipping a beat, "piped-up" and listed all the items on the list. She told me, at that time, it didn't even register to her that he remembered all the items. In the past, he had the better memory, and on this occasion, she didn't think this was so different. Only later did it occur to her that this was an unusual event. She then made the connection between the antibiotics and her husband's ability to remember on that day.

During a later appointment, long after the antibiotic therapy had ended, I noticed that Albert was having trouble keeping his teeth clean. I also noticed a deterioration of Mary's hygiene as well. I tried to encourage her to help Albert with his hygiene; however, she said she was so depressed with Albert's condition she had started to drown it all in alcohol. She just couldn't face the task. At that appointment, a microscopic examination revealed a spirochetal infection in her mouth, as well, for the first time. She was very discouraged to hear that news. I felt very helpless in their situation. These people needed help, but as a dentist, I couldn't give it to them.

It has been awhile since they have come back to my office. Efforts to get them to return for follow-up treatment have failed. Here is a situation that might be best treated in the same fashion as Lyme disease, long-term antibiotic treatment for both of them. I can treat the periodontal disease, but need cooperation from the patients every day for their hygiene. These patients are far down the road to not being able to care for themselves. If the theory presented in this book proves to be true, then early treatment of periodontal disease (oral spirochetosis) may have avoided this condition altogether. Mary and Albert did not deserve the miserable condition they've found themselves at the end of life. They should be enjoying retirement and life in general, not having to deal with Alzheimer's disease and its devastating effect on their lives.

Parkinson's Disease Case: Several months ago, David, a 45-year-old Caucasian male with Parkinson's disease, presented to my office for implant treatment. He had many missing teeth because of periodontal disease and several decayed remaining teeth.

Parkinson's disease is a progressive disorder of the central nervous system. It causes tremors (especially in the hands) and rigidity (especially in the face). The disease affects men and women equally, primarily after age 60. However, approximately 10 percent of those with the disease are under age 40. Although no cure for the disease is available at this time, drug therapy can help alleviate the symptoms.

I did a microscopic examination on David and found a spirochetal infection. I put him on the Life Guard program and got his periodontal condition under control. I also restored the multiple decayed teeth. It has been several months and he is ready to continue his implant treatment.

I was curious to see if his Parkinson's disease symptoms had showed any improvement as a result of my periodontal treatment. He indicated that it had. He said, "I had extreme difficulty putting a seatbelt on in my car. Now I can easily put it on." I know that periodontal treatment won't cure Parkinson's or any other neurological condition; however, by eliminating the source of the suspected bacteria that might be the cause, at least the condition won't deteriorate further. I gave this patient no encouragement that it would. This observation is anecdotal, but time will tell if the correlations hold up in future research. It is noteworthy that this chronic neurologically diseased Parkinson's patient also had oral spirochetes, similar to Albert, the previous patient with Alzheimer's disease.

<u>Fibromyalgia Case:</u> Six months ago, Susan, a 35-year-old Hispanic female, came to my office for implant dentistry. She reported a history of fibromyalgia.

Fibromyalgia, also called FMS, makes one feel tired and causes muscle pain and "tender points." Tender points are places on the neck, shoulders, back, hips, arms or legs that are sensitive to touch. People with fibromyalgia may have other symptoms, including trouble sleeping, morning stiffness, headaches, and problems with thinking and memory, sometimes called "fibro fog." These are all symptoms of chronic Lyme disease as well.

No one knows what causes fibromyalgia. Anyone can get it, but it is most common in middle-aged women. People with rheumatoid arthritis and other autoimmune diseases, also symptoms of Lyme disease, are particularly likely to develop fibromyalgia. There is no cure for fibromyalgia, but medicines can help manage symptoms. Getting enough sleep and exercising may also help.

Susan had all of the above symptoms and was discouraged with her condition. She had lost many teeth because of periodontal disease and felt that if she could get her gum disease under control and replace some of her missing teeth she would feel better about herself. During the diagnosis procedure I did a microscopic examination and found a severe spirochetal infection in her periodontal tissue.

Is this a coincidence that this patient with fibromyalgia, who exhibits symptoms similar to Lyme disease, also has oral spirochetosis? Why are all these people with spirochetes in general complaining about the same symptoms? Is there a correlation? I researched what is known about fibromyalgia. Unfortunately, not much is known and it seems to be a "catch all" for diseases, such as this, when no definitive diagnosis can be found. In the face of Lyme disease–like symptoms, it was not surprising to me to find microscopic evidence of oral spirochetosis, a spirochetal infection in her mouth.

I put her on the Life Guard program to treat her periodontal disease. In her particular case, I used the CO_2 laser to eliminate the lining of the gingival sulcus. She had tooth sensitivity, as I did extra fluoride irrigations around her teeth at the gumline.

This patient responded particularly well to the treatment. Though I was not treating her fibromyalgia, when I finished her periodontal treatment, which took about two months, I enquired as to how she felt physically. She related to me that she felt substantially better. Her life seemed to come back into her. She laughed and joked with us, and I noticed a vast improvement in her general demeanor and vitality of her skin tone.

Her periodontal condition is ready for dental implants. During the next months, we will complete her treatment by replacing her missing teeth. Again, it is noteworthy that this is one more chronic inflammatory disease that I found an active spirochetal infection in the gingival sulcus.

Skin Conditions That Remarkably Improved After Periodontal Treatment: All of the above described patients had great improvement of the color and the look of vitality of their skin tone. They just looked healthier. The next three patients were very remarkable and even my staff mentioned to me that they saw the difference once the periodontal treatment was completed.

One year ago, Jennifer, a 65-year-old Caucasian female, presented to my office for a consultation on dental implants. She looked much older than her age. She had blotched, discolored skin, the look of poor health and slow deliberate speech. She was missing most of her teeth but wanted to save as many of the remaining teeth as possible. Jennifer told me her life story that day. Her father was a poor estate gardener who married his boss—the widow and benefactor of an extremely rich San Diego philanthropist. This famous person donated generously to charities. She told me she could get the money needed for her dental treatment from her stepmother.

During the normal source of diagnosis and treatment planning, I took a microscopic sample of her plaque and viewed it under the microscope. She had a spirochetal infection. I put Jennifer on the Life Guard program. Within weeks of her treatment, her blotched skin disappeared and she regained her normal color and skin texture. It was so remarkable that everyone in my office noticed the drastic change. The patient was elated.

During that time she approached her stepmother for funding the implant treatment. Her stepmother gave her a loan for the Life Guard treatment but refused to pay for her implants.

I thought that this woman, whose husband had generously given to establish medical facilities in San Diego, would be interested in funding a PBS documentary about my research. So I sent her one of the earlier drafts of this book and a letter describing the improvement of her stepdaughter's skin condition. She declined in a personal letter back to me and then proceeded to criticize my hand-written signature. She did thank me for helping her step-daughter's skin condition, which after many attempts, no other doctor had been able to do. Maybe after the book comes out and she reads it again, she will have more positive thoughts.

Nine months age, Patricia, a 53-year-old Philippine female and the mother of a friend, presented to my office for an implant dentistry consultation. She had many missing teeth because of periodontal disease. A microscopic examination revealed a spiro-chetal infection. She was placed on the Life Guard program, and several weeks later, her infection was under control. Implants were then placed.

Patricia responded well to her treatment, and within a short period of time, her skin appeared radiant—in comparison to the dry, aging appearance she initially presented. Both her daughter and Patricia were impressed by the remarkable improvement.

Kim, a 35-year-old Vietnamese female, presented to my office for an implant dentistry consultation. During the examination process, I found she had a very active spirochetal infection. She had severe acne on her face, particularly around her mouth. I placed her on the Life Guard program. Because of the severity of her periodontal situation, it took two rounds of treatment to resolve her periodontal condition.

The one most remarkable improvement was the condition of her acne. It completely cleared. This was the serendipity of her peri-odontal treatment. So many patients' skin condition improves once the oral bacteria is brought under control.

Summary

The more I understand periodontal disease and the consequences of oral spirochetosis, the more I observe the relationships between it and systemic disease in my periodontal diseased patients. I believe I am just scratching the surface of this problem. More research is needed and more funds need to be made available to further study this relationship.

APPENDICES

Appendix I

*"**Endarteritis Obliterans:** Endarteritis is an inflammation of the internal coat of an artery or capillary, generally of chronic type. Its pathogeny is as follows: In direct contact with the blood is the endothelium (a layer of flattened cells); next is the tunica intima, composed of elastic fibers arranged longitudinally; next comes the middle coat, composed of muscular fibers arranged transversely. The outer coat consists of longitudinal connective tissue, which contains the vasa vasorum. In the capillaries, the intima lies in immediate contact with the surrounding tissue, or accompanied by a rudimentary advertitia. In other words, the walls of the capillaries consist of almost nothing but the intima. The capillaries have certain contractibility; they contract or dilate without muscular fibers. The veins probably also have a certain amount of contraction and dilation from irritability of the intima. Each coat of the arteries takes on special types of inflammation. The causes of endarteritis are numerous. Inflammation of the intima of the blood vessels may be due to irritation from without or within.*

When it occurs from without, any local irritation will set up an inflammation that may extend to the outer coats of the capillaries. This produces a marked increase of blood. The vasa vasorum becomes swollen; the white blood corpuscles crowd into the terminal capillaries and migrate into the extra vascular spaces. Rapid proliferation of the round-cell elements takes place. The walls of the vessels become thickened. Owing to the projecting intervals of the intima, the caliber of the blood vessel diminishes.

Irritation occurring from within, results either from trophic changes in the system from direct irritation from toxaemias, or from both interdependently. Under these circumstances, a germ disease or other toxins may have an affinity for a certain organ, tissue or part, and produce irritation in the capillaries in a distant part of the body."

This was quoted word for word from the old textbook written by Eugene S. Talbot, MD DDS[93] in 1899.

Appendix II

The following are expanded descriptions of the case studies which I presented earlier in the book. The below descriptions contain unabridged details not found in the text of this book.

CASE #1:

A thirty-seven-year-old woman of Vietnamese descent received three implants, in order to replace a missing molar and bicuspid tooth. Within months after the implants were completed, approximately three millimeters of bone loss occurred around the top of these contiguously placed dental implants. The bone loss was predominantly caused by a spirochetal infestation of the crestal bone area, which was diagnosed by observing a plaque sample taken from the infected site and viewing it under a microscope at a magnification of 1000X . Plaque samples examined from other gum sulci areas in this patient's mouth revealed the presence of similar spirochetal bacteria. At the onset of, and during treatment, the patient never exhibited any traditional signs or symptoms of periodontal disease. I also observed that the patient had excellent oral hygiene. After discovering the spirochetal infection, the patient was treated systemically with antibiotics for two weeks. During the second week, while the patient was still on antibiotics, I performed an ultrasonic scaling and teeth cleaning on her. All gingival sulci were irrigated with Chlorohexidine (0.12%)[94]. I then performed a revision surgery to remove the threads and polish the implants that were exposed above the bone. Follow-up examinations of the plaque samples showed no re-infestation of the bacteria.

CASE #2:

A fifty-four-year-old man with periodontal disease had his upper teeth extracted and a custom implant placed. Over the next twelve years, episodes of infection would occur around the upper implant, and these were treated with various antibiotics; however, the infections always returned. During those years, and without the aid of a microscope, I did not know whether the patient was getting re-infected from some outside source, or whether indigenous bacteria were causing the infections. In 2007, I performed bacterial studies on his tissue with the use of a microscope. The results revealed a spirochete infection. I placed the patient on antibiotics (500 milligrams of Metronidazole and 500 milligrams of amoxicillin, three times per day for two weeks) and we scheduled a visit for the implant to be removed. At the end of the two weeks, the patient requested, if at all possible, to save the implant.

I then performed another microscopic examination of his gum tissue and concluded that the antibiotic regimen had not killed the spirochetes, because they had, over the years, somehow developed resistance to the drugs. A culture of this plaque was taken at that time and sent to the University of Southern California microbiology laboratory for testing. The implant was then removed.

The microbiological laboratory reported that several types of bacteria had survived the antibiotic treatment: namely, p. intermedia, t. forsythia, campylobacter and fusobacteria species, and enteric gram-negative rods. The report indicated that no Treponema denticola were present, even though microscopically, spirochetes had been visually present at the time that the sample was taken. This evidence indicated that the spirochetes, whatever they were, had developed resistance to the powerful antibiotics used to eradicate them, and had survived the treatments even though the culture revealed no spirochetes. The spirochetes, however, were not the Treponema denticola type that the laboratory had tested for, but rather unknown types which couldn't be tested for.

In addition, microscopic evidence of multiple spore spherical bodies and granular forms were found after antibiotic treatment. They appeared as dense granular doughnut- shaped substances surrounded by a white halo, with a hollow light refractive center. Such forms were identical to those described in the medical literature.

After the patient was given antibiotics, I performed an evaluation on him using a microscope, which revealed morphological candidates for the cystic form of spirochetal bacteria. This discovery further supports evidence that oral spirochetes have similar survival strategies to other types of spirochetes; namely, those of Lyme disease and syphilis.

CASE #3:

A forty-three-year-old woman came into my office for an implant treatment. She had periodontal disease and bone loss and spirochetes were identified microscopically. I treated her with antibiotics, following the same regimen as the above cases; however, because of stomach problems, she wasn't able to complete the regimen. I extracted several of her teeth and placed implants in 2001, and periodically examined her over the next several years. At her most recent follow-up examination (in 2007), I discovered severe bone loss on one natural tooth #12 adjacent to bone loss on an implant. On the contra-lateral side of her mouth, I also observed seven to eight millimeters of bone loss from two adjacent implants. Examination of her dental plaque with a microscope revealed the presence of a spirochete infection. I once again placed her on antibiotics and removed the single infected tooth #12 and adjacent implant. The other two implants were treated and saved. I removed and microscopically examined the granulation tissue (infected tissue) from around the two implants, and found that it was loaded with spirochetes throughout. Notice the large ball or cystic form with many spiro-chetes connected to, spinning furiously and pointing concentrically away from its surface, as if trying to escape from the structure to which they are attached. From my observations, I concluded that spirochetes were the reason for this patient's implant failure. I performed a follow-up microscopic examination a week later, amidst the patient's two-week antibiotic treatment regimen, and again found spherical, spore forms similar to those discovered in the previous case.

CASE #4:

A forty-five-year-old woman came into my office with periodontal disease. Her condition required a tooth extraction and an implant placement. This patient had a history of five failed periodontal surgeries over the past twenty years. A microscopic examination of her dental plaque revealed a severe spirochete infection. As the patient in the previous case, this patient's large spirochetes were found to be in the form of large cysts, and loaded with granular material. Several hundred large spirochetes surrounded these cyst-like structures and seemed to be attached to them (as possibly some sort of colony of spirochetes). After observing the Borrelia cyst forms pictured in MacDonald's Lyme disease research, I realized that the cystic structure of this patient's spirochetes was very similar, if not identical, to that of MacDonald's description. I placed my patient on antibiotics (500 milligrams of Metronidazole and 500 milligrams of amoxicillin, three times per day for two weeks) and re-examined her one week later. Under the microscope, I observed that granular and cystic forms of the bacteria were still present; however, I did not find any active spirochetes. As in the previous two cases, there were numerous spores with the same white halo, hollow light-refractive center and dense, grainy-appearing material.

Appendix III

EDITOR'S NOTE: Dr. Nordquist has recently been conducting in vitro experiments which aim to expose oral spirochetes to electromagnetic fields in an attempt to observe whether or not these fields can kill the bacteria. Experiments of this type have been conducted in the past, namely, by Doug MacLean, inventor of the "Doug Coil Machine" (see http://www.lymeandrifebook.com for more information).

However, past experiments have been frustrating due to the elusive nature of spirochete infections found throughout the body. Oral spirochetes are easier to observe than other types of systemic spirochetes. Doug MacLean did not have access to oral spirochetes. Hence, Dr. Nordquist's research may be very valuable, and may present new data which has never before been available.

To learn more about this area of research, visit:

Dr. Nordquist's Blog:
http://www.biomedpublishers.com/nordquist

Bryan Rosner's book explaining research history:
http://www.lymeandrifebook.com

Endnote Citations

[1] Center for Disease Control and Prevention (CDC): Center for Disease Control and Prevention. http:www.cds.gov/nccdphp/aag_cvd.htm.

[2] Albert et al. An examination of periodontal treatment and per member per month (PMPM) medical costs in an insured population. BMC Health Services Research 2006, 6:103. or http://www.biomedcentral.com/1472-6963/6/103.

[3] http://www.pbs.org/wgbh/takeonestep/heart/

[4] Ellen R, Galimanas V. Spirochetes at the forefront of periodontal infections. Periodontology 2000. 2005:38(1);13-32.

[5] www.pbs.org/wgbh/takeonestep/heart

[6] Beck JD et al. Periodontitis: a risk factor for coronary heart disease? Ann Periodontol. 1998;3(1):127-41

[7] Jodhpur K et al. Strength of evidence linking oral conditions and systemic diseases. Commend Cetin Educe Dent Supply. 2000;(30):12-23.

[8] Jodhpur KJ et al. Possible explanations for the tooth loss and cardiovascular disease relationship. Ann Periodontol. 1998;3(1):175-83.

[9] DeStefano F et al. Dental disease and risk of Coronary heart disease and mortality. BMJ 1993;306:688-992.

[10] Loesche WJ et al. Periodontal disease as a risk factor for heart disease. 1994 Compend Contin Educ Dent;25(8):976-992.

[11] Loesche WJ et al. Periodontal disease: link to cardiovascular disease. 2000;21(6):463-6, 468, 470 passim.

[12] Behle JH, Papapanou PN. Periodontal infections and atherosclerotic vascular disease: an update. 2006;56(4 Suppl 1):256-62.

[13] Geerts SO et al. Further evidence of the association between periodontal conditions and coronary artery disease. J Periodol;75(9):1274-80.

[14] Scannapieco FA Position paper of the American Academy of Periodontology: periodontal disease as a potential risk factor for systemic diseases. J Periodol 1998;69(7):841-50.

[15] www.nidcr.nih.gov/AboutNIDCR/SurgeonGeneral/ExecutiveSummary.htm

[16] Riviere GR et al. Molecular and immunological evidence of oral Treponema in the human brain and their association with Alzheimer's disease. Oral Microbiol Immunol. 2002;17:113-118.

[17] Harvey LF. Loosening of the teeth. Advertiser. 1869-70;I:73-79.

[18] Discussion of Riggs' disease: Its diagnosis and treatment. Conn Vall Dent Soc Trans. 1874:93-94.

[19] Mills GA. More about Rigg's disease. Amer J Dent Sci. 1880-81;14(3):143-144.

[20] Witzel A, The treatment of Pyorrhoea alveolaris, or Infectious Alveolitis. Advertiser(Dental). 1883;24:139-145.

[21] Pyorrhoea Alveolaris treated by Riggs. Advertiser(dental). 1885;24:41-43.

[22] Kilker CH. The relationship of Vincent's organism to pyorrhea Alveolaris. Summary. 1920;XL:496-499.

[23] Socransky SS, Haffajee AD. Evidence of bacterial etiology: a historic perspective. Periodontology 2000. 1994;5:7-25.

[24] Watson MR, Bretz WA, Loesche WJ. Presence of Treponema denticola and Porphyromonas gingivalis in children correlated with periodontal disease of the parents. J Dent Res. 1994;73(1):16-40.

[25] Lee Y, Tchaou WS, Loesche WJ. The transmission of BANA-positive bacterial species from caregivers to children. J Am Dent Assoc. 2006;137(11):1539-46.

[26] Lee Y et al. The transmission of anaerobic periodontopathic organisms. J Dent Res;85(2):182-6.

[27] Jacquet L Sezary A. Des formes atypiquees et degeneratives du treponeme pale. 1907 Bull Soc Med HSP Paris 4:114-116.

[28] Hindle E On the life-cycle of Spirochaeta gallinarum. 1912 Parasitology;4:463-477.

[29] Mattman LH. Cell wall deficient Forms, 3rd ed. CRC Press 2001.

[30] Pam Weintraub, Cure Unknown, St. Martin's Press, June 2008

[31] Oksi J et al. Borrelia burgdorferi detected by culture and PCR in clinical relapse of disseminated Lyme borreliosis, Ann Med. 1999;31(3):225-32.

[32] Coyle PK. Neurologic complications of Lyme disease. Rheum Dis Clin North Am. 1993:19(4):993-1009.

[33] MacDonald A. Plaques of Alzheimer's disease originate from cysts of Borrelia Burdorferi. The Lyme disease spirochete. Elsevier Editorial system for Medical Hypothesses. 2006 Manuscript Number YMEHY-D-06-00134R1.

[34] Personal phone conversation with Alan MacDonald. 05-11-2007.

[35] Farrell GM, Martin EH. Borrelia burgdorferi: another cause of food borne illness? Int J Food Microbiol. 1991 Dec;14(3-4):247-60.

[36] Rosner B. The Top 10 Lyme Disease Treatments 2007 BioMed Publishing Group.

[37] Smithe K, Riviere H. Molecular and immunological evidence of oral Treponemas in the human brain and their association with Alzheimer's disease. Oral Mico Imm. 2002:17;113-118.

[38] Miklossy J. Alzheimer's disease-a spirochetosis? Neuroeport,1993 Jul:4(7):841-8.

[39] Desal HG, Gill HH, Shankaran PR, Mehta PR, Prabhu SR. Dental Plaque: A Permanent Reservoir of Helibacter pylori. Scand J Gastroenterol 1991;26:1205-1208.

[40] Brorson O, Brorson S. An in vitro study of the susceptibility of mobile and cystic forms of Borrelia Burgdorferi to Metronidazole. APMIS 1999:107(6):566-576.

[41] http://www.lymenet.de/literature/cystsl.htm

[42] Nishida M et al. Dietary vitamin C and the risk for periodontal disease. 2000 J Periodontol;71(8):1215-23.

[43] Melville TH, Slack GL. Bacteriology for Dental Students. 1960 William Hienemann Medical Books:pg.170.

[44] Wolf V, Lange R. Weeks J. Development of quasi-multicellular bodies of Treponema denticola. Arch Microbiol;1993:160:206-213.

[45] De Ciccio A, McLaughlin R, Chan C. Factors affecting the formation of spherical bodies in the spirochete Treponema denticola. Oral Microbiol Immunol 1999:14(6);384-386.

[46] Becker W, Becker B, Newman M, Nyman S. Clinical and microbiological findings that may contribute to dental implant failures. Int J Oral Maxillofac Implants 1990;5:31-38.

[47] Rosenberg E, Torosian J, Slots J. Microbial differences in 2 clinically distinct types of failures of osseointegrated implants. Clin Oral Implant Res 1991;2:135-144.

[48] Mombelli A, Van Oosten M, Schurch E, Lang N. The microbiota associated with successful or failing osseointegrated titanium implants. Oral Microbiol Immunol 1987;2:145-151.

[49] Riviere G, DeRouen T, Kay S, Avera S, Stouffer V Hawkins N. Association of oral spirochetes from sites of periodontal health with development of periodontitis. J Periodontol 1997;68:1210-1214.

[50] Farrell GM, Marth EH. Borrelia burgdorferi: another food borne illness? Int J Food Microbiol. 1991 Dec;14(3-4):247-60.

[51] Choi BK et al. Spirochetes from digital dermatitis lesions in cattle are closely related to treponemas associated with human periodontitis. Int J Syst Bacteriol. 1997 Jan;47(1):175-81.

[52] Colligham RJ et al. A spirochete isolate from a case of severe virulent ovine foot disease is closely related to a Treponema isolated from human periodontitis and bovine digital dermatitis. Vet Microbiol 2000 Jun 1;74(3):249-57.

[53] Demirkan I et al. Serological evidence of spirochaetal infections associated with digital dermatitis in dairy cattle. Vet J. 1999 Jan;157(1):69-77.

[54] Edwards AM et al. From tooth to hoof: Treponemas in tissue-destructive diseases.
J Appl Microbiol. 2003;94(5):767-80.

[55] Mattman L. Cell Wall Deficient Forms 2001 CRC Press LLC 61-62.

[56] Personal conversation.

[57] Xavier K, Bassler B. LuxS quorum sensing: more than just a numbers game. Curr Opin Microbiol 2003 apr;6(2):191-7.

[58] Federie M, Bassler B. Interspecies communication in bacteria. J Clinical Invest. 2003 nov;112(9):1291-9.

[59] Miller S, Xavier K, Campagna S, Taga M, Semmelhack M Bassler B, Hughson F. Salmonella typhimurium recognizes a chemical distinct form of bacterial quorum-sensing signal AL-2. Mol Cell 2004 Sep 10;15(5):677-87.

[60] Chen et al. Structural identification of a bacterial quorum-sensing signal containing boron. Nature. 2002 Jan;31;415(6871):488-9.

[61] Camilli A, Bassler B. Bacterial small signaling pathways. Scienc. 2006 Feb 24;311(5764)1113-6.

[62] Lens D, Bassler B. The small nucleoid protein Fis is involed in Vibrio cholerae quorum sensing. Mol Microbiol. 2007 Feb;63(3):859-71.

[63] Lens et al. CsrA and three redundant small RNAs regulate quorum sensing in Vibrio cholae. Mol Microbiol. 2005 Nov;58(4):1186-202.

[64] Tseng C, Chen Y, Pang I, Weber H. Peri-implant pathology caused by periapical lesion of an adjacent natural tooth: a case report. Int J Oral Maxillofac Implants 2005;20(4):632-5.

[65] Brisman D, Brisman B, Moses M. Implant failures associated with asymptomatic endodontically treated teeth. JADA 2001;132(Feb)191-195.

[66] Yip K, Mui M, Newsome P, Chow T, Sham A. Assessment of endodontically treated teeth adjacent to proposed implant sites. Implant Dentistry 2002;11(4):349-353.

[67] Scarano A, Domizio P, Petrone G, Lezzi G, Piattelli A. Implant periapical lesion: A clinical and Histologic case report. J Oral Implantol 2000;26(2):109-113.

[68] Shaffer M, Juruaz D, Haggerty P. The effect of periredicular endodontic pathosis on the apical region of adjacent implants. Oral surg Oral Med Oral Pathol Radiol Endol 1998;86(5):578-81.

[69] Sussman H. Periapical implant pathology. J Oral Implantol 1998;24(3):133-38.

[70] Sussman H. Cortical bone resorption secondary to endodontic-implant pathology. A case report. N Y State J 1997 Nov;63(9):38-40.

[71] Sussman H. Implant pathology associated with loss of periapical seal of adjacent tooth: clinical report. Implant Dent 1997;6(1):33-7.

[72] Sussman H, Moss S. Localized osteomyelitis secondary to endodontic-implant pathosis. A case report. J Periodontol 1993; 64(4):306-10.

[73] Brynolf I. A histological and roentgenological study of the periapical region of upper incisors. Odont Revy. 1967;(11):1-97.

[74] Green T, Walton R, Merrell P. Radiographic and histologic periapical findings of root canal treated teeth in cadaver. Oral surg Oral Med Oral Pathol Radiol Endol 1997;83:707-11.

[75] Peters LB et al. The fate and role of bacteria left in root dentinal tubules. 1995 Int Endod J;28(2):95-9.

[76] Blaylock RL. Inflammation: The real cause of most diseases. Vol.5 No. 6, 2008.

[77] Elter JR, Champague CM, Offenbacbacter S, Beck JD. Relationship of periodontal disease and tooth loss to prevalence of coronary heart disease. J Periodontol. 2004;75(6):782-90.

[78] Okoro CA et al. Tooth loss and heart disease: findings from the Behavioral Rich Factor Surveillance System. 2005 Am J Prev Med;29(5 Suppl 1):50-6.

[79] Ylostalo PV et al. Gingivitis, dental caries and tooth loss: risk factors for cardiovascular diseases or indicators of elevated health risks. 2000 J Clin Periodol;33(2):92-101.

[80] Holmlung A. et al. Severity of periodontal disease and number of remaining teeth are related to the prevalence of myocardial infarction and hypertension in a study based on 4,254 subjects. 2006 J Periodol;77(7):1173-8.

[81] Panagakos FS, Volpe AR, Petrone JD, DeVizio W, Davies RM. Advance oral Antibacterial/Anti-inflammatory Technology: A Comprehensive Review of the Clinical Benefits of Triclosan/Copolymer/Fluoride Dentifrice. J Clin Dent. 2005;16(Supplement):S1-S20.

[82] Tonetti MS et al. Treatment of Periodontitis and Endothelial Function. 2007 N Engl J Med;356(9):911-20.

[83] Nordquist WD. The Effect of Prior Acid Etch on the Rate of Sn3F3PO4 Formation Subsequent to Topical SnF2 Treatment, Master of Science Thesis, University of Louisville 1973.

[84] Harper DS, Loesche WJ. Inhibition of acid production from oral bacteria by fluorapatite-derived fluoride. J Dent Res 1986 Jan;65(1):30-3.

[85] Huges CA, Yotis WW. Effect of fluoride on Treponema denticola. Infect Immun. 1986 Jun;52(3):914-5.

[86] Li YH, Bowden GH. The effect of environmental Ph and fluoride from the substratum on the development of biofilms on selected oral bacteria. J Dent Res. 1994 Oct;73(10):1615-26.

[87] Love RM, Jenkinson HF Invasion of dentinal tubules by oral bacteria. Department of Stomalogy, University of Otago School of Dentistry, PO Box 647, Dnmedin, New Zealand.

[88] Nordquist W.D, Krutchkoff DJ. Investigation of the Sub-surface Reaction Phase with Prolonged SnF2-Enamel Interaction. 1973 ;IADR:203.

[89] Nordquist WD, Krutchkoff DJ. Effect of Prior Acid Etch on the Rate of Sn3F3PO4 Formation Subsequent to Topical SnF2 Treatment. 1973;IADR;697: 233.

[90] Nordquist WD, Krutchkoff DJ, Wei SHY. Effect of Prior Acid Etch on the Rate of Sn3F3PO4 Formation Subsequent to SnF2 Topical Treatment. J Dent Res1975.

[91] Nordquist WD, Krutchkoff DJ, Wei S.H.Y. Morphology and Kinetics of the Sn3F3PO4 Crystal Growth on Human Enamel Slabs Subsequent to SnF2 Treatment. J. Dent. Res., 1975.

[92] Mazza JE et al. Clinical and antimicrobial effect of stannous fluoride on periodontitis. J Clin Periodontol. 1982;8(3):203-12.

[93] Talbot ES. Interstitial Gingivitis or so-called pyorrhea alveolaris. The SS White Dental Manufacturing Co. 1899.

[94] Slots J, Winkelhoff A. Antimicrobial therapy in periodontics. CDA Journal 1993;21(11);51-56.

Breinigsville, PA USA
25 February 2010
233193BV00001B/40/P